MW00413211

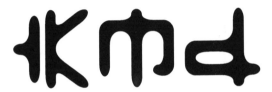

Ketogenic Mediterranean Diet

Please visit us on the Internet
to find updated information, answers to
frequently asked questions, printable documents
(e.g., grocery shopping list, daily logs), and more:

http://AdvancedMediterraneanDiet.com

Join the discussion at Dr. Parker's blogs:

http://AdvancedMediterraneanDiet.com/blog/
http://DiabeticMediterraneanDiet.com
http://PaleoDiabetic.com

Also by Steve Parker, M.D.:

*Advanced Mediterranean Diet: Lose Weight, Feel
Better, Live Longer*
*Conquer Diabetes and Prediabetes: The Low-Carb
Mediterranean Diet*

Dr. Parker's current research interest is application
of the Paleolithic diet as therapy for diabetes.

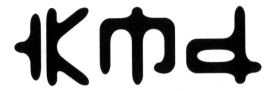

Ketogenic Mediterranean Diet

Steve Parker, M.D.

pxHealth

Copyright © 2012 by Steve Parker

All rights reserved. No part of this book may be repro-
duced or transmitted in any form or by any means without the prior written permission of the author, except for
the inclusion of brief quotations in critical articles and
reviews.

First edition published 2012
ISBN 978-0-9791284-2-4
Library of Congress Control Number: 2011917822

Published by pxHealth
PO Box 27276
Scottsdale, Arizona 85255 USA
Web: http://pxHealth.com

Cover by Brian Parker Lee
http://BrianParkerLee.com

Publisher's Cataloging-in-Publication data

Parker, Steven Paul.
    KMD : Ketogenic Mediterranean diet / Steve Parker,
M.D.
        p. cm.
        ISBN 978-0-9791284-2-4
        Includes bibliographical references and index.

1. Diet --Mediterranean Region. 2. Cooking, Mediterranean. 3. Weight loss. 4. Diet therapy --Mediterranean Region. 5. Obesity --Prevention 6. Insulin resistance --Diet
therapy. 7. Low-carbohydrate diet. 8. Dietary Carbohydrates --Administration & dosage --Popular Works. I.
Title.

RM222.2 .P37 2012
613.2/5 –dc22   2011917822

CONTENTS

Dedicated to my patients

Disclaimer

The ideas and suggestions in this book are provided as general educational information only and should not be construed as medical advice or care. All matters regarding your health require supervision by a personal physician or other appropriate health professional familiar with your current health status. Always consult your personal physician before making any dietary or exercise changes. The publisher and author disclaim any liability or warranties of any kind arising directly or indirectly from the use of the Ketogenic Mediterranean Diet. If any problems develop, always consult your personal physician. Only your physician can provide you medical advice.

The names in patients' cases discussed herein have been changed to protect their identities.

Introduction

Medical and nutrition scientists have made several watershed advances in our understanding of optimal nutrition and weight management over the last decade.

The most astounding new finding is that the saturated fat and total fat content of our diets does not cause or contribute to heart and vascular disease. The same is true for cholesterol in our food. In other words, foods that contain fat, saturated fat, and cholesterol don't cause us to have heart attacks, strokes, or hardening of the arteries (atherosclerosis), or high blood pressure. These statements apply to a large majority of people, although there may be rare exceptions.

This new knowledge, which is accepted by most experts in medical nutrition science, runs counter to popular thought and teaching of the last four decades. At the same time, it's true that the information hasn't yet trickled down to many physicians and dietitians working in the trenches of clinical care. The scientific supporting literature is listed at the back of the book in the Selected References section.

The second eye-opening development is the discovery that certain carbohydrates are particularly prone to make us gain excess fat weight, and that avoiding those carbohydrates can be especially helpful in weight management. This is best demonstrated by numerous scientific studies that document more successful weight loss in dieters who drastically reduce consumption of carbohydrates, at least for the short term. The idea that carbohydrates are uniquely fattening applies to a majority of people, but certainly not all. The scientific supporting literature is listed at the back of the book in the Selected References section.

A third groundbreaking scientific discovery in recent years involves the role of physical activity in weight loss. To lose excess weight, you've got to exercise a lot, right? That's now old school thought, and not really true. The latest research tells us that, in general, exercise contributes only minimally to successful real-world weight loss. "Real world" as opposed to The Biggest Loser TV show. How much does exercise contribute to weight-loss? Only about 10%. What about exercise's role in long-term weight management and prevention of weight regain? That's a whole 'nother can o' worms.

These advances led me to design a very-low-carbohydrate version of the Mediterranean diet—the Ketogenic Mediterranean Diet—for loss of excess weight. It may eventually prove useful for management of seizures, certain tumors, and neurodegenerative disorders, but I cannot yet recommend it for those purposes.

The book you hold, to a large extent, is an abridgement of my *Advanced Mediterranean Diet* (second edition), with a focus on very-low-carb eating.

Nutrition experts have long recognized the Mediterranean diet as the healthiest way of eating for the general public, particularly those not struggling with excess weight or diabetes.

The traditional Mediterranean diet is rich in olive oil, fresh fruits and vegetables, nuts, fish, wine, whole grains, cheese, and yogurt, with minimal red meat. It's heavily influenced by the cuisines of Greece and southern Italy.

MEDITERRANEAN DIET HEALTH BENEFITS

Strong evidence supports the Mediterranean diet's association with:
- increased life span
- lower rates of cardiovascular disease such as heart attacks and strokes
- lower rates of cancer (prostate, breast, uterus, colon)
- lower rates of dementia
- lower incidence of type 2 diabetes

Weaker supporting evidence links the Mediterranean diet with:
- slowed progression of dementia

- prevention of melanoma (serious skin cancer)
- lower severity of type 2 diabetes, as judged by diabetic drug usage and blood sugar levels
- less risk of developing obesity
- better blood pressure control in the elderly
- improved weight loss and weight control in type 2 diabetics
- improved control of asthma
- reduced risk of developing diabetes after heart attack
- reduced risk of mild cognitive impairment
- prolonged life of Alzheimer disease patients
- lower rates and severity of chronic obstructive pulmonary disease lower risk of gastric (stomach) cancer
- less risk of macular degeneration
- less Parkinson's disease
- increased chance of pregnancy in women undergoing fertility treatment
- reduced prevalence of metabolic syndrome (when supplemented with nuts)
- lower incidence of asthma and allergy-like symptoms in children of women who followed the Mediterranean diet while pregnant

MEDITERRANEAN DIET IN DETAIL

So what exactly is the traditional, healthy "Mediterranean diet"? Here are the predominant features:
- it maximizes natural whole foods and minimizes highly processed ones
- small amounts of red meat
- less than four eggs per week
- low to moderate amounts of poultry and fish
- daily fresh fruit

- seasonal locally grown foods with minimal processing
- concentrated sugars only a few times per week
- wine in low to moderate amounts, and usually taken at mealtimes
- milk products (mainly cheese and yogurt) in low to moderate amounts
- olive oil as the predominant fat
- abundance of foods from plants: vegetables, fruits, beans, potatoes, nuts, seeds, breads and other whole grain products
- naturally low in saturated fat, trans fats, and cholesterol
- naturally high in fiber, phytonutrients, vitamins (e.g., folate), antioxidants, and minerals (especially when compared with concentrated, refined starches and sugars in a modern Western diet)
- naturally high in monounsaturated and polyunsaturated fats, particularly as a replacement for saturated fats

So, what's wrong with Mediterranean-style eating if you're overweight or diabetic? Those fattening carbohydrates I mentioned previously. The Mediterranean diet typically derives over half its calories from carbohydrates. The Ketogenic Mediterranean Diet limits the fattening carbohydrates while retaining the healthy ones.

IF YOU HAVE DIABETES

Many people with diabetes are taking medications that can drop blood sugar levels dangerously low. They can still follow the Ketogenic Mediterranean Diet, but must have close medical supervision and adjustment of drug dosages. I discuss this issue and many other diabetes-related topics in *Conquer Diabetes and Prediabetes: The Low-Carb Mediterranean Diet*. Diabetics should not attempt the Ketogenic Mediterranean diet without benefit of that book.

THE KEY TO WEIGHT MANAGEMENT: KNOWLEDGE

I will assume that you're overweight and reading this book to lose weight. My goal is to share with you the information that has helped my personal patients lose weight effectively, safely, and permanently. Reduction of excess body fat has been particularly critical for my patients with high blood pressure, heart problems, diabetes, strokes, low back pain, and lower limb arthritis. Even if you're essentially healthy, you may need to lose 10 to 50 pounds (4.5 to 23 kg) in order to feel and look your best.

The standard medical approach to weight loss too often is:

- a five-minute lecture on proper eating and exercise habits
- presentation of a confusing, unrealistic, calorie-restricted diet pamphlet
- occasional referral to a dietitian
- follow-up office visits with focus more on the medical problem than the weight problem.

But this approach nearly always fails, and those few who do lose weight typically regain it within a few weeks or months. The reasons for failure of weight loss programs are numerous and complex, but they share a unifying characteristic: lack of knowledge.

We need adequate knowledge of nutrition and how our bodies work to avoid wasting time, money, and energy on worthless weight-loss schemes. We must learn to easily identify weight-loss plans that are designed only to enrich the entrepreneur. We must learn to recognize scams that may jeopardize our physical and emotional health. Most importantly, knowledge is your key to successful long-term weight management. Given an adequate knowledge base, most people don't need to consult physicians, dietitians, or other advisers on weight loss.

Acquisition of that knowledge base, however, is not easy. Information and opinions are readily available from the Internet, books, television, magazine and newspaper articles, friends and acquaintances, health food store clerks, hearsay at the beauty salon, and advertisements for various weight-loss products. Much of this is worthwhile, much is worthless.

How do you separate the wheat from the chaff? The "doctor" in my doctor of medicine degree is based on the Latin word for "teacher." I'll share with you what your personal up-to-date physician likely would teach you, if only he had the time. He would help you find the pearls of knowledge in a sea of complexity, confusion, contradiction, and quackery. My aim is to educate you so that you can seize control of your weight problem.

Although some of the information presented here is common knowledge, most of it is gleaned from my three decades of clinical experience with overweight patients and from my analysis of scientific literature generated by obesity researchers and clinicians.

The scientific literature is neither readily available nor understandable to the layperson. Furthermore, technical popularizers in the media tend to sensationalize preliminary research results. They may unwittingly promote fads since they lack the scientific training and clinical experience to recognize the real, but rare, breakthroughs. Having observed my patients' weight-loss efforts of every description, I know what works and what doesn't.

ACKNOWLEDGEMENTS

Sir Isaac Newton wrote in 1676: "If I have seen further, it is by standing on the shoulders of giants." He was acknowledging that his scientific success had been built upon the achievements of other scientists. While no one would ever mistake me for a Newton, I am similarly indebted to generations of scientists and physicians who have discovered and shared basic truths in the fields of nutrition, physiology, pathophysiology, and epidemiology. These are the foundations of this book.

I am grateful to Linda Kimmel, medical librarian, for her help acquiring the scientific literature, and to Scottsdale Healthcare for funding her position. I am obliged to innumerable dietitians and nutritionists who generously shared their knowledge with me. I am indebted to my patients, who helped me learn the art and science of medicine through the privilege of caring for them. Thanks to Art Chance for his participation years ago in our two-man think tank dedicated to improving health through exercise and nutrition.

Certain individuals have influenced my ideas about nutrition and fitness over the last few years in a positive way. A partial list (in no particular order) includes Monica Reinagel, Jimmy Moore, Regina Wilshire, Dave Dixon, Douglas Robb, Gary Taubes,

Michael R. Eades, Robert C. Atkins, Laura Dolson, Lyle McDonald, Dr. J, Emily Deans, Tom Naughton, Beth Mazur, Sandy Szwarc, Travis Saunders, Peter Janiszewski, Richard David Feinman, Skyler Tanner, Darya Pino, Alex Hutchinson, K. Dunn Gifford, Yoni Freedhoff, Stephan Guyenet, Amy Dungan, Richard K. Bernstein, Arya M. Sharma, Dan Buettner, Conner Middelmann-Whitney, Jennifer Eloff, Eric Westman, Stephen Phinney, and Jeff Volek. I'm grateful to them for having stimulated my cerebral synapses. Any errors in this book are strictly mine, not theirs.

I thank my immediate family (Sunny, Dan, Brian, Casey, Paul, and Austin) for enduring my nutritional obsession, including recurrent dinner-table discussions of junk food, whole grains, calories, carbohydrates, and fiber. I am especially indebted to my wife for her role as steadfast supporter, sounding board, and Mediterranean chef. I love you, Sweet Pea. I thank God for enabling me to present this information to you. Any good that comes from it is from Him.

The second day of a diet is always easier than the first. By the second day you're off it.

— Jackie Gleason

There are no secrets to success. It is the result of preparation, hard work, learning from failure.

— General Colin Powell

1

What Causes Overweight and Obesity?

"I've become my mother!" cried Janice as she studied her reflection in a full-length mirror on her 40th birthday. She had ballooned from 130 to 175 pounds (59 to 80 kg) over the last 15 years. Janice didn't think twice about her weight until after her first baby, Ashley, was born when Janice was 24. She gained 30 pounds (14 kg) during the pregnancy, but was down 15 pounds (6.8 kg) by the time she left the hospital. The other 15 pounds, which she called baby fat, hung around. During her teen years, Janice had been active in her school's marching band and regularly played softball. She jogged two or three miles a couple days per week, just to keep in shape for her beloved softball.

After Ashley was born, Janice still played softball, but couldn't find the time to jog. Her second child, James, was born two years after Ashley. Household life began to get hectic. Janice's husband was working 60-hour weeks at the tire store. Her mother, 40 pounds (18 kg) overweight, remarked how hard it was to chase Ashley around the house when she babysat. Janice decided to table softball until the kids were older.

Janice added another eight pounds of lingering baby fat while pregnant with James. She got a job at a call center six months after his birth. She sat most of the day, processing orders for various products. The family's evening meal, by necessity it seemed, was too often a sack of fast food she picked up on the way home. Janice didn't have the time or energy for exercise after cleaning, shopping, and laundering. She drank four cans of Dr. Pepper every day for the pleasure and a boost of energy.

The surgeon who removed Janice's gallstones at age 35 told her they were caused by her excess weight. She began to worry about other health effects and her lack of energy and stamina. Years after giving up softball, she tried jogging around the block just once and strained her right hamstring muscle. No more jogging for her, she decided.

Over the next five years, Janice tried many of the popular diets: low-fat, Atkins, cabbage soup, Nutri-System, Jenny Craig. They all worked great. For a while. She lost eight to 15 pounds (6.8 kg) , then lost her enthusiasm. Two months later she would be back up to her baseline weight, if not higher.

Since breast cancer runs in her family, Janice came to me for a routine physical and referral for a mammogram. At the end of our visit, she asked, almost as an afterthought, "Hey, doc, what can I do to get this weight off?" It was the end of my workday so we had time to chat. She shared her frustration with her prior weight-loss efforts. She told me her dream of fitting into some of her old clothes and wondered if her husband would ever again look at her the way he did when they were newlyweds. She mentioned the stress and time constraints of a two-teenager household, and how the teens would eat only two kinds of food: fast food and junk food. She told me how it hurt when she had to turn down the school's request to chaperone her son's four-mile nature hike with his class; she knew she just didn't have the stamina.

I shared with Janice my own frustration in dealing with my patients' medical problems that were caused or clearly aggravated by their excess weight. I saw hundreds of patients like Janice give their honest and best efforts to lose weight and keep it off, only to fail. Their medical problems were good for my business, but I longed for better outcomes for my patients. I had seen weight-loss methods of all kinds come and go, then come again. Surely, there had to be a better way. I vowed to review the situation comprehensively, to learn definitively what we should be eating and doing, and to share with Janice the results of my efforts. In these pages, you'll see what I discovered.

BASIC STATS

Sixty-six percent of adults in the United States are chubby, pudgy, portly, plump, rotund, stout, corpulent, or just plain fat. These adjectives fall somewhere on the spectrum from mildly overweight to morbidly obese. Overweight means having more adipose tissue (commonly known as fat) than is considered healthy or normal by historical standards. Obesity refers to the more extreme accumulations of fat. Of the 66% of us who are overweight or obese, about half are overweight and half are obese.

A healthy weight for a 5-foot, 4-inch person (163 cm) would be 108 to 145 pounds (49 to 66 kg) ; obesity starts at 175 pounds (79.5 kg). For someone 5-foot, 10-inches tall (178 cm), a healthy weight is 128 to 174 pounds (58 to 79 kg), with obesity starting at 208 pounds (94.5 kg).

Have you ever noticed in old photographs how everyone seemed so skinny, even gaunt? The pictures don't lie. In fact, photos tend to make us look heavier. Despite a barrage of popular media reports touting exercise, healthy lifestyles, and low-fat eating, the prevalence of adult obesity in the United States increased from 13% of us in 1960 to 34% in 2010. That's one in three.

And our children (ages 6–19) are learning by example: 19%—one in five kids—are now overweight, gradually rising over the last three decades.

About 30% of United States men and 45% of women are dieting currently, either in pursuit of culturally ideal attractiveness or health and longevity.

WHAT CAUSES OVERWEIGHT?

It's complicated. I don't want to bore you with too many details, so here's a simplified explanation.

Overweight can be defined simply as excessive storage of energy in the form of fat. To some extent, it's the result of an imbalance between energy intake and energy expenditure. Energy intake is food. Energy expenditure is a combination of physical activity and metabolism.

Metabolism refers to the complex chemical and physical processes in our bodies that are necessary for the maintenance of life. In metabolism, some substances are broken down to produce energy for vital processes, such as breathing, blood circulation, and generation of body heat. The other side of metabolism is formation of vital substances and structures, as in tissue repair or blood production. When more energy (food) is put into the system than is necessary for metabolism and physical activity, the excess is stored as fat. That fat is available to produce energy just as the wax in a candle is burned to release its stored energy as light and heat. Indeed, some candles are made from fats (tallow).

The fine balance between energy intake and expenditure is influenced by numerous factors, including heredity, environment, psychology, and basic physiologic mechanisms.

INSULIN: THE FAT-BUILDING HORMONE

Insulin is a major hormone influencing fat accumulation. In response to eating carbohydrates (and proteins to a much lesser extent), the pancreas secretes insulin into the bloodstream to lower blood sugar levels that rise in response to digestion of carbohydrates. If we eat too many carbohydrates, the resulting blood sugar will be converted to fat tissue. Eating fewer carbohydrates lowers the amount of circulating insulin, which could help with weight management. More on this later.

HEREDITY

Studies documenting an association between heredity and obesity have lead to unnecessary discouragement of dieters. If your genes totally determine your degree of fatness, it would indeed be a waste of time fighting heredity. Accept your fate and pig out! But genes are only a piece of the puzzle. Note that Japanese-American men living in Hawaii and California are 15 pounds (6.8 kg) heavier and two to three times more likely to become obese than are their counterparts remaining in Japan. Furthermore, the prevalence of obesity in the United States has doubled since 1900. These data speak more in favor of environmental and cultural influences since the gene pool does not change nearly that fast.

AGING

In the United States, both men and women tend to gain excess fat weight from early adulthood to middle age, with body weight peaking around age 50 or 60. Doubtless, we tend to be less physically active as we get older, and therefore "burn" fewer calories (units of energy). It's also true that the rate of metabolism slows by 2% per decade in adulthood. If food intake doesn't diminish comparably, weight gain results. One-third of us are able to buck the weight gain trend.

ANCESTRY AND THE THRIFTY GENE HYPOTHESIS

Throughout most of human history, mere survival required a great expenditure of energy in the form of physical activity. Our forebears struggled to find and collect food, build shelter, and make clothing. Firewood for heat, cooking, and light was gathered piece by piece. Potable water was not available at simply the flick of a wrist.

In prehistoric days, abundant food was available sporadically and seasonally, if at all. Lacking refrigeration or other effective means of food storage, our ancestors gorged when they had the chance. Their goal was storage of food energy in the one place available to all: fat tissue. Those who could store more energy (fat) were more likely to survive the hardscrabble times when food was scarce due to poor weather, wildfires, disease, and competition. Survivors had genes that facilitated fat storage. For better or worse, they passed these genes down to us.

With the advent of the Neolithic Agricultural Revolution some 10,000 years ago, we became less dependent on the whims of nature. Crop cultivation yielded a steadier and larger supply of food while requiring less work. A few individuals, now with a bit of free time and excess energy, began the development of the arts, philosophy, music, science, and technology.

The Industrial Revolution of the late 18th century then freed the rest of us (in the developed world) from the constant, energy-draining struggle for mere survival. Scientific and technological advances afforded us the basic necessities of life with less physical labor. In 1900, well over two-thirds of the American work force was in farming; today fewer than 2% of us farm. Individuals can now expend yet more effort on intellectual pursuits, such as expansion of our knowledge base and further technological advances. We even have the time and energy for stamp collecting, surfing, bird watching, facebooking, fiddling, TV watching, and other such frivolities.

Whereas our ancestors spent untold hours and energy gathering fruit and berries or hunting game, we have labor-saving devices that wash our dishes and change our TV channel for us. Imagine how much more energy we would expend if not for refrigeration, plumbing, electricity, cars, computers, and telephones! As more machines and technology do our work, we require less food energy (calories). In reality, Americans eat more calories than we did 30 years ago.

In a nutshell, our increasingly prevalent overweight problem stems from a biological predisposition to store excess energy as fat, coupled with our sedentary lifestyles and abundant food. Compared to our Paleolithic ancestors, we have incredible access to grains, concentrated sugars, and vegetable or seed oils (such as corn and soybean oil).

If we just look at the last 100 years, we find our diets in the U.S. have changed dramatically. For example, refined sugar consumption in the U.S. was 11 lb (5 kg) in the 1830s, rising to 155 lb (70 kg) by 2000. Over the last 30 years in the U.S., consumption of sugar-sweetened beverages has increased from 3.9% of total calories to 9.2%. In that same time span, the percentage of overweight or obese American adults increased from 47% to 66%. The obesity percentage alone rose from 15 to 34% of adults.

Furthermore, soybean oil consumption increased from essentially zero a century ago to 7.4% of total calories today. Check the ingredients on processed food labels and there's a good chance you'll find soybean oil.

A RADICAL THEORY OF OBESITY FROM GARY TAUBES

At the start of my medical career three decades ago, many of my overweight patients were convinced they had a hormone problem causing it. I carefully explained that's rarely the case. As it turns out, I may have been wrong. And the hormone is insulin.

Science writer Gary Taubes has popularized what I'll call the "carbohydrate/insulin theory of obesity" in his 2007 masterpiece, *Good Calories, Bad Calories*. For details, the average consumer is better off reading his 2011 book, *Why We Get Fat*.

Mr. Taubes says, "We don't get fat because we overeat; we overeat because we're getting fat." Read that again and let it sink in. We need to think of obesity, says Taubes, as a disorder of excess fat accumulation, then ask why the fat tissue isn't regulated properly. A limited number of hormones and enzymes regulate fat storage; what's the problem with them?

Mr. Taubes makes a great effort to convince us the old "energy balance equation" doesn't apply to fat storage. You remember the equation: eat too many calories and you get fat, or fail to burn up enough calories with metabolism and exercise, and you get fat. To lose fat, eat less and exercise more. He prefers to call this the "calories-in/calories-out" theory. He admits it has at least a little validity. Problem is, the theory seems to have an awfully high failure rate when applied to weight management over the long run. We've operated under that theory for the last half century, but keep getting fatter and fatter. So the theory must be wrong on the face of it, right? Is there a better one?

Here is Taubes' explanation. The hormone in charge of fat storage is insulin; it works to make us fatter, building fat tissue. If you've got too much fat, you must have too much insulin action. And what drives insulin secretion from your pancreas? Dietary carbohydrates, especially refined carbs such as sugars, flour, cereal grains, starchy vegetables (e.g., corn, beans, rice, potatoes), and liquid carbohydrates. These are the "fattening carbs." Dozens of enzymes and hormones are at play either depositing fat into tissue, or mobilizing the fat to be used as energy. It's an active process going on continuously. Any regulatory derangement that favors fat accumulation will *cause* gluttony (overeating) or sloth (inactivity). So it's not your fault.

If Taubes Is Right, How Do We Lose Excess Fat?

Cut back on carb consumption to lower your fat-producing insulin levels, and you turn fat accumulation into fat mobilization. Especially avoid the "fattening carbs."

Before you write off Taubes as a fly-by-night crackpot, be aware that he's received three Science-in-Society Journalism Awards from the National Association of Science Writers. He's a respected, professional science writer. Having read two of his books, it's clear to me he's very intelligent. If he's got a hidden agenda, it's well hidden.

One example illustrates how hormones control growth of tissues, including fat tissue. Consider the transformation of a skinny 11-year-old girl into a voluptuous woman of 18. Various hormones make her grow and accumulate fat in the places we now see curves. The hormones make her eat more, and they control the final product. The girl has no choice. Same with our adult fat tissue, but with different hormones. If some derangement is making us grow fatter, it's going to make us more sedentary (so more energy can be diverted to fat tissue) or make us overeat, or both. We can't fight it. At not least very well, as you can readily appreciate if look at the people around you at any American shopping mall.

If cutting carbohydrate consumption is so critical for long-term weight control, why is it that so many different diets—with no focus on carb restriction—seem to work, if only for the short run? Taubes suggests it's because nearly all diets reduce carbohydrate consumption to some degree, including the fattening carbs. If you reduce your total daily calories by 500, for example, many of those calories will be from carbohydrates. Simply deciding to "eat healthy" works for some people: stopping soda pop, candy bars, cookies, desserts, beer, etc. That cuts a lot of fattening carbs right there.

Losing excess weight or controlling weight by avoiding carbohydrates was the conventional wisdom prior to 1960, as documented by Mr. Taubes. Low-carb diets for obesity date back almost 200 years. The author attributes many of his ideas to German internist Gustav von Bergmann (1908).

Taubes rejects the calories-in/calories-out theory of overweight that hasn't done a very good job for us over the last 40 years. Taubes' alternative ideas deserve serious consideration.

STRAIGHT UP, DOC . . . WHY AM I FAT?

Remember that insulin is the major fat-building hormone, and carbohydrates are the main cause of insulin release from the pancreas. Refined starches and concentrated sugars in particular raise insulin output. Overweight in advanced countries is usually caused by excessive consumption of these fattening carbohydrates.

A LOOK AHEAD

Recall that overweight results from an imbalance between energy intake and energy expenditure. You must overcome this imbalance if you're to lose weight.

By the time you finish this book, you'll have the facts and motivation you need to lose your excess weight and keep it under control for the long run. We'll briefly review physiology and nutrition, then explore the consequences of obesity and the benefits of exercise in more depth. Only then will you be ready for my eating plan for successful weight loss. Finally, I'll tell you how to be successful at the most troublesome, frustrating, and mysterious area of weight control: long-term maintenance of weight loss.

KEY POINTS

- 66% of U.S. adults are overweight or obese.
- Fat is stored energy.
- We have a biological predisposition to store excess energy (calories) as fat. Sedentary lifestyles and abundant food contribute to fat storage.
- Insulin is the primary fat storage hormone.
- Overweight in advanced countries is usually caused by excessive consumption of fattening carbohydrates such as refined starches and concentrated sugars.

- Gary Taubes' "carbohydrate/insulin theory of obesity" is a major advancement in current thinking about the cause of overweight.

I went into a McDonald's yesterday and said, "I'd like some fries." The girl at the counter said, "Would you like some fries with that?"

— Jay Leno

Success is the sum of small efforts, repeated day in and day out...

— Robert Collier

2

Why We Eat
and What Happens Next

"Would you like fries with that?" the clerk asked Tom after he ordered a Big Mac, apple pie, and chocolate shake at the drive-thru. He was already salivating. "Sure, why not?" Tom didn't realize, or care, that he had just ordered 1,770 calories, which is about what many people eat in an entire day. Tom eats three meals a day. It sure tasted good.

Tom grew up in a small Texas town. At age 17 he was 6-feet, 2-inches (188 cm) tall and large enough to help take his high school football team to the state championship playoff his junior and senior years. Football reigned supreme on Friday nights back in those days, not only for Tom, but the entire town. With weightlifting and football practice, Tom was exercising about three hours on most days and eating 5,000 to 6,000 calories. He didn't call it exercise, it was just who he was. He remembers often washing down an apple pie with a quart of milk in one sitting. Yes, the whole pie.

Like his father, Tom was a meat-and-potatoes kind of guy who ignored most fruits and vegetables. That was rabbit food. His favorite meal was slow-cooked barbecue brisket, potato salad, and baked beans flavored with brown sugar and bacon. Tom's wife, Barbara, knew that the men in his family were prone to overweight, heart attacks, high blood pressure, and high cholesterol. Tom stubbornly resisted her gentle pressure to eat healthier, whatever that meant. Eating was about enjoyment, in his mind, not about what his body needed.

Tom was a passable student and earned a football scholarship at a Texas college. A severe knee injury at the end of his sophomore season put the kibosh on his dreams of a pro football career and sidelined him for a good year while healing. He had always loved working with his hands, so he dropped out of college to become a full-time carpenter. His bosses at the construction company eventually rewarded his management skills by making him a supervisor. After that, he did less physical labor, but worked more hours. In his 30s, Tom still enjoyed the Friday night football games. But now he was sitting in the stands sipping sodas and chowing down on corndogs. He wasn't exercising three hours a day anymore, but he could still finish off a whole pie in a day. His only exercise was an occasional trip to the park to play catch with his young son.

Tom's father had his first heart attack at age 59, when Tom was 37. Dad had seemed the picture of health, except for the spare tire around his middle. Reality assaulted Tom with the fact that Dad might not always be around. Tom even thought about changing some of his own health habits. He heard all about the diet and lifestyle changes recommended by his father's doctors. Barbara made sure of that! But Dad recovered and Tom put health concerns on the back burner.

Six months later, Tom started having chest pains right behind the breastbone. His first thought was, "Oh, no! Is this what a heart attack feels like?" He couldn't have a heart attack at age 37, could he? Typical for a man, Tom ignored it as best he could. The first pains resolved spontaneously. The later pains seemed to improve with Maalox or Tylenol. But the pains got worse and more frequent. It was getting harder to hide it from Barbara.

During a particularly bad spell, he broke into a cold sweat as his heart palpitated. Realizing how bad off he was, he wondered if he would be around to see his son grow up. That's when he admitted he better get some professional help and a life insurance policy. Calling 911 was definitely the right thing to do. He let Barbara make the call, then he was admitted to my service at the hospital.

Tom was lucky. Tests showed he was only suffering from an unusually bad case of heartburn; stomach acid was irritating his esophagus. We could manage that condition with medication and diet changes, but his eating habits were sending him a warning. I shared with him my sense that he was headed toward an early heart attack, like his father. His eat-whatever-tastes-good diet, high blood pressure (154/100 mm/Hg)), high cholesterol (250 mg/dl or 6.5 mmol/l), high triglycerides (310 mg/dl or 3.5 mmol/l), sedentary ways, and his weight all added up to an unhealthy lifestyle. His "game weight" at age 20 was 220 pounds (100kg), all muscle and bone. Now he was 308 pounds (140 kg), with much less muscle. Tom's encounter with his own mortality accomplished what his wife's health-conscious exhortations could not. He was now ready to make major lifestyle changes, and asked for my guidance.

PHYSIOLOGY, NUTRITION, AND WEIGHT LOSS

If you have absolutely no interest in science or how your body runs, skip the rest of this chapter.

To lose your excess fat safely and permanently, you must understand how you acquired it in the first place and how fat tissue fits in with other components of your body. We need to review some basic principles of physiology and nutrition.

Physiology is the branch of biology dealing with the functions and vital processes of organisms or their parts and organs. Nutrients are substances in food that are used in the body to provide energy and structural materials, and to regulate the growth, maintenance, and repair of the body's tissues. Nutrition as a science is the study of nutrients in foods and of the body's handling of them in processes necessary for life, growth, and optimal health.

The commercial success of worthless weight-loss scams is testament that many people are relatively ignorant of nutrition and physiology. Some have forgotten what they once learned. Others are subject to wishful thinking or delusion. Many want to believe that weight loss is easy, that a session with a hypnotist will do the trick, that a vitamin and herb mix will "melt away the fat," that weight-loss pills alone are a safe long-term solution, that they can eat anything they want if they are in the right program. But wishing does not make it so.

There are six major classes of substances, called nutrients, that the body uses for growth, maintenance, and repair of tissues. They are water, fat, protein, carbohydrates, vitamins, and minerals.

A healthy 140-pound (64 kg) body contains about 85 pounds (39 kg) of water and 25 pounds (11 kg) of fat. The remaining 30 pounds (14 kg) are mostly protein, carbohydrate, and the bone minerals: calcium and phosphorus. All other minerals and vitamins together weigh less than a pound (0.5 kg).

Your body can make some nutrients for itself. But there are at least 40 specific nutrients, each one essential for health, that you can obtain only from food. Eating the right foods is critical.

WATER

Without water, there is no life as we know it. The sum of chemical and physical processes necessary for the maintenance of life is called metabolism. Nearly all these processes occur in, or are dependent on, water. Life is a myriad of chemical reactions mostly occurring inside cells. Cells are the smallest living structural units capable of independent functioning. Millions of cells of different types are joined together to form our various tissues and organs. In addition to participating in many chemical reactions, water transports various vital materials (such as vitamins, minerals, sugar, amino acids) within and between cells. Water carries waste products away from cells.

A healthy body is 55–60% water. On average, we lose three to four cups (800 ml) of water per day through sweating and breathing (water vapor). Also, the kidneys must produce at minimum two cups

35

(480 ml) of urine daily to carry away waste products. We must replace these obligatory water losses. Water balance is carefully regulated by interactions between the brain (hypothalamus, pituitary), kidneys, adrenal glands, mouth, and stomach.

Water is so important that we can only live a couple weeks without it.

FAT

For too long, dietary fat has been demonized as bad for us. In fact, it has many wonderful attributes as a component of our diets and bodies. As a nutrient, it provides us with fat-soluble vitamins (A, D, E, and K), enhances food flavor, and provides building blocks for cell structures (e.g., cell membranes) and hormones. Moreover, dietary fat is a great source of inexpensive energy. As part of our bodies, fat provides insulation to conserve heat, provides shock absorption and cushioning (e.g., the buttocks), and stores huge amounts of energy. In the sphere of human relations, sufficient fat in the right places is essential to physical attractiveness.

TERMINOLOGY OF FATS

"Fat" can refer to all three types of lipids: triglycerides, sterols, and phospholipids. But usually fat refers to triglycerides, which make up 99% of stored body fat.

Triglycerides are composed of carbon, oxygen, and hydrogen atoms arranged as a molecule of glycerol with three fatty acids attached. A fatty acid is a chain of carbon atoms with attached hydrogens and an acid group at one end.

Carbon atoms must have four bonds with adjacent atoms. A fatty acid carrying the maximum possible number of hydrogen atoms is "saturated." Red meat typically is high in saturated fatty acids. If a couple of adjacent hydrogen atoms are missing, the two side-by-side carbon atoms in the chain form a double bond.

A fatty acid with one double bond and two hydrogen atoms missing is a "monounsaturated fatty acid," such as oleic acid. Olive oil has lots of monounsaturated fatty acids such as oleic acid.

A fatty acid with two or more carbon double bonds (and four or more missing hydrogens) is "polyunsaturated," such as linolenic or linoleic acid. Most vegetable oils fit this description.

Vegetable and fish oils have an abundance of polyunsaturated fats. Olive and canola oils are rich in monounsaturates. The tropical oils are an exception. Despite plant origins, coconut and palm oils are primarily saturated.

Food manufacturers can synthesize fats by adding hydrogen to the carbon-to-carbon double bonds in liquid vegetable oils. Food labels often refer to these artificial fats as hydrogenated or partially hydrogenated vegetable oils, trans fats, or trans-fatty acids. "Trans" refers to the altered three-dimensional configuration of the new molecule.

A triglyceride is formed when the acid ends of three fatty acids attach to glycerol. Triglycerides usually contain mixtures of fatty acids with variable carbon chain lengths and degrees of saturation. Fats and oils are overwhelmingly (95%) triglycerides.

There are two fatty acids that we need but our bodies cannot make: linoleic and linolenic acid. Nutritionists call these "essential fatty acids" since we must eat them for optimal nutrition and, indeed, for life. We can make other fatty acids by combining two-carbon fragments derived from carbohydrates, protein, and alcohol. The new fatty acids attach to glycerol, forming triglycerides which can be taken up by adipose cells. This is how excessive intake of non-fat nutrients, especially carbohydrates, leads to overweight.

In addition to triglycerides, there are two other types of lipids: sterols and phospholipids. Well-known sterols are cholesterol, vitamin D, sex hormones, bile acids, and cortisol. They share a basic structure of carbon, oxygen, and hydrogen arranged in multiple rings.

Sterols in food are a minor source of calories. Our bodies synthesize the sterols we need for metabolic processes. For example, the liver manufactures the cholesterol that becomes a major component of new cell walls. Over 90% of total body cholesterol is tied up in cell walls.

Phospholipids have a structure similar to triglycerides but contain a few atoms of phosphorus and nitrogen. They serve primarily as cell wall components.

DO DIETARY FATS CAUSE HEART DISEASE?

Until just recently, physicians thought that dietary fat and saturated fats in particular were a major cause of atherosclerosis, also known as hardening of the arteries. The hardening isn't so bad; the problem is that it's accompanied by obstructive plaque in the walls of arteries. The plaque impairs the flow of blood to vital tissues, and the plaque can rupture, allowing the sudden formation of a blood clot that stops all blood flow. Tissue downstream from the clot dies. So atherosclerosis is the cause of most heart attacks, strokes, and poor circulation. It also contributes to high blood pressure.

The American Heart Association in 1957 recommended that polyunsaturated fats replace saturated fats in an effort to reduce heart and vascular disease. U.S. public health recommendations in 1977 were to reduce fat intake to 30% of total calories to lower the risk of coronary heart disease (atherosclerosis of the heart arteries). Slowly, some fats were replaced mostly with carbohydrates, highly refined ones at that. This shift tends to raise blood triglycerides and lower HDL cholesterol levels, which may themselves contribute to atherosclerosis. Current recommendations are, essentially, to keep saturated fatty acid consumption as low as possible.

The latest scientific evidence, however, indicates that total dietary fat and saturated fat have little, if anything, to do with causing atherosclerosis, heart attacks, strokes, or poor circulation in most people. (For details, see Selected References at the end of the book.) In fact, replacing dietary fats with carbohydrates may have contributed significantly to the steady rise in overweight and obesity we've seen over the last forty years in the U.S.

Trans fats, however, are still thought to contribute to heart and vascular disease. Food manufacturers using these man-made fats continue to reduce utilization in response to public pressure and concern. A safe minimal level of consumption has never been established.

DIGESTION AND UTILIZATION OF FATS

After a meal, digestive juices inside the small intestine go to work on ingested fats (triglycerides), removing two or all three of the fatty acids from the glycerol molecule. The resulting pieces are absorbed by cells lining the small intestine, where they are reassembled into triglycerides. These new triglycerides are pumped into the bloodstream and circulate all over the body to be used either as an immediate source of energy or stored in fat tissue as a future energy supply. Fat cells pluck any excess triglycerides from blood and store them as a glob of fat.

Later, when other cells need fuel energy, fat cells break down the triglycerides and kick fatty acids and glycerol into the bloodstream. The energy-starved cells pick up these triglyceride fragments and break them down further in chemical reactions that ultimately yield carbon dioxide, water, and energy.

Thanks to fat stores, a person of average weight can survive up to two months of total starvation. A fatter person can survive even longer.

PROTEIN

Proteins are complex chains of amino acids that play vital roles:
- in growth, replacement, and repair of all tissues
- as enzymes regulating chemical processes
- as antibodies fighting infection
- in fluid balance
- in acid-base balance
- as hormones (e.g., insulin, thyroid

hormone)
- in blood clotting
- as an emergency energy source when carbohydrates and fats are limited.

Amino acids have a central carbon atom with four attachments: a hydrogen atom, an amino group, an acid group, and a variable side group or side chain. The 20 common amino acids are distinguished by their individual side groups.

Most proteins are composed of between 20 to several hundred amino acid building blocks linked together chain-like in a specific sequence. Chains of amino acids may also be linked together, often via sulfur atoms, to form even larger complex molecules. For instance, insulin consists of a specific sequence of 51 amino acids in two chains linked by sulfur bridges.

Food digestion breaks down dietary protein into its component amino acids, which we then use to make the proteins we need. If not available from the diet, our bodies can synthesize 11 of the 20 common amino acids.

But there are nine amino acids that we cannot make and must obtain from food. These are referred to as "essential amino acids." If not in the diet, the body will break down its own proteins to obtain these essential amino acids. Avoid this self-cannibalism by eating the right foods!

Formation of protein in a cell requires that all the needed amino acids be available simultaneously. Non-essential amino acids are pulled out of the circulating pool or manufactured right in the cell. But if the diet supplies too little of an essential amino acid, protein synthesis will be limited. Over time, the result is malnutrition.

A "complete protein" food contains all nine of the essential amino acids, in about the right proportions as humans require. Proteins in foods from animals (poultry, fish, meat, eggs, cheese, and milk) are generally complete. Eggs and milk contain particularly high-quality proteins.

Plant-derived foods provide less protein per unit of measure, and tend to be deficient in one or more essential amino acids. Soy protein, however, is complete and is sometimes used as a meat replacement. Vegetarians who exclude all animal-derived foods can receive all the amino acids they need if they eat a variety of legumes, grains, vegetables, nuts, and seeds (e.g., sunflower, sesame). The idea is to combine two or more foods so that the essential amino acids missing from one are supplied by the other.

For healthy adults, the protein Recommended Dietary Allowance is 0.8 grams per kilogram of appropriate body weight per day. This is about 50 grams for an average-sized person. As examples, a slice of bread has three grams of protein, a cup (240 ml) of milk has eight grams, a cup of beans has 13 grams, three ounces (84 g) of meat has 21 grams of protein. We in the United States generally eat much more protein than needed.

CARBOHYDRATES

Carbohydrates mainly serve as a source of energy for us, providing about half of the energy in the standard American diet. The other half comes mostly from fat. Relatively little of our energy comes from protein.

There are essential amino acids (in proteins) and there are essential fatty acids (in fats): "essential" meaning our bodies cannot make them so we must eat them for life and health. There are no essential carbohydrates; we can make the ones we need.

Carbohydrates are made only of carbon, oxygen, and hydrogen.

The most fundamental carbohydrate is a simple sugar called glucose. It's used as an energy source by all the cells in our body. It's like the gasoline needed to run a car, a car that's always running. Although we eat relatively little pure glucose, most dietary carbohydrates are converted during digestion to glucose, which is used as fuel. Any excess glucose not needed immediately for energy is converted to a storage form, called glycogen, for later use. We have the capacity to store only a half day's worth of energy in glycogen. Carbohydrates are converted to fat when eaten in excess of what we can use immediately as energy or store as glycogen.

The preceding paragraph is exceedingly important for anyone with an excess weight problem. Read it again.

Carbohydrates are composed of sugars. Basic sugar molecules contain six carbon atoms, twelve hydrogen atoms, and six oxygen atoms. The various atoms are arranged in simple structures to form the three most basic sugars: glucose, fructose, and galactose. These ring-like structures are called monosaccharides.

When a chemical reaction joins a pair of monosaccharides together, the result is a disaccharide. The one most familiar to you is sucrose, or table sugar.

Sucrose, lactose, and maltose are the three most important disaccharides. Each of them has a glucose ring molecule attached to a ring of fructose, galactose, or another glucose. Lactose is the major carbohydrate in milk, contributing up to 50 percent of its calories. The monosaccharides and disaccharides are "simple carbohydrates," also called sugars.

"Complex carbohydrates" are much larger molecules composed of straight or branched chains of linked monosaccharides, mostly glucose. The three important complex carbohydrates, also known as polysaccharides, are starch, glycogen, and fiber.

Starch is a storage form of energy in plants. Through photosynthesis, green plants use sunlight's energy to form carbohydrates from carbon dioxide and water. Carbohydrates not used as structural parts of the plant can be stored as glucose chains, i.e., starch. After planting, the starch in a grain of corn supplies energy to the seedling until it can capture sunlight's energy through its leaves. Starchy foods such as wheat, rice, potatoes, and legumes provide not only energy but potentially a wealth of vitamins, minerals, and other healthful substances if they are not removed by processing.

Glycogen is a storage form of energy in animals. It's composed of numerous glucose molecules tied together in highly branched chains. In contrast, starch chains in plants are unbranched or only occasionally branched. Glycogen and starch are otherwise so similar that glycogen is sometimes referred to as animal starch. One third of total body glycogen is in the liver, two thirds is in muscle tissue. Muscle is stingy, tending to hold onto glycogen-glucose for its own use. On the other hand, a major function of the liver is to rapidly breakdown glycogen and release glucose into the bloodstream whenever another tissue needs energy.

Fibers are mostly complex carbohydrates forming the structural parts of plants. Cellulose is a good example since it's the primary structural element of all plant cell walls and you're familiar with it as a component of paper. Human digestive enzymes cannot break down the types of bonds between fiber monosaccharide units. Fiber passes undigested through the small intestine, but bacteria in the large intestine partially digest it. This benefits the bacteria and we get a few short-chain fatty acids in the bargain.

Eating too much dietary fiber can cause intestinal discomfort and gas, and may interfere with absorption of some nutrients (e.g., minerals). Fiber may be so filling that it displaces other necessary nutrients that we might have eaten if not full. That's not a big worry, though. Inadequate fiber intake is much more prevalent and may have adverse health consequences. The potential health benefits of high dietary fiber intake include:

- lower blood cholesterol
- improved blood glucose levels in diabetics
- improved weight control
- prevention of constipation, hemorrhoids, and diverticulosis

DIGESTION AND UTILIZATION OF CARBOHYDRATES

When you eat a baked potato or bowl of rice, chewing stimulates the salivary glands to secrete an enzyme that starts breaking down complex carbohydrates into smaller polysaccharides. But the small intestine does the bulk of the digestive work; chemical reactions governed by enzymes disassemble starches and disaccharide sugars down to mono-saccharide units (glucose, fructose, and galactose). Monosaccharides are absorbed into the blood and flow downstream to the liver, where fructose and galactose are converted to glucose.

At this point you have a hefty load of glucose in the liver and must "decide" what to do with it. There are only two choices: kick it back into the bloodstream for distribution to energy-hungry cells, or store it as energy to use later. If you're already overweight, you want to store it as glycogen instead of fat, or burn it up as an energy source right now.

One of the liver's major functions is to store glucose (as glycogen) and release it as needed. Cells need a constant energy supply and can get that energy from glucose or fat. Some tissues, most notably the brain and nerves, are almost entirely dependent on glucose as their energy source. Cells take glucose out of circulation and split it into smaller fragments, yielding energy, carbon dioxide, and water.

Even when cells use fat for energy they still need some glucose for the most efficient utilization of fat.

Our bodies have elaborate mechanisms for maintaining blood glucose at an optimal range (about 70–140 milligrams per deciliter or 3.9–7.8 mmol/l) so that cells, particularly in the brain and nerves, don't "run out of gas." Blood glucose falling too low triggers the breakdown of glycogen into glucose, which the liver pumps into the bloodstream.

Just how much glucose is circulating in our blood-streams anyway? In a normal, healthy state, not much: about a teaspoon (5 ml).

While fat tissue stores enough energy to last for weeks, we can only store enough glycogen to last a matter of hours. When it is gone, the body can produce significant amounts of glucose only by disassembling proteins or fats.

Your body just isn't able to convert much fat into glucose. Remember that fats are triglycerides: three fatty acid chains attached to a small glycerol molecule. You can convert the glycerol into glucose, but glycerol is only 5% of the fat molecule. The fatty acids can be broken down through a process called fatty acid oxidation, producing energy, but not glucose. Our bodies can also make limited amounts of glucose from dietary protein or by breaking down our own body proteins.

So the glucose your body craves as immediate fuel usually comes from daily dietary carbohydrates, or from the limited glycogen stored in your body.

What happens if you drastically reduce your consumption of carbohydrates for days on end? Where do your cells get the energy needed to survive and thrive? They get most of it from your body fat stores, which break down to fatty acids and glycerol. The fatty acids are metabolized (oxidized) to supply energy to most tissues. Glycerol and proteins provide the glucose needed by the brain and nerves.

This switch in energy metabolism from one based on carbohdyrates to one based on fats is how, for example, people can live for a couple months without any food whatsoever. It also explains how we sleep through a long night and skip occasional meals without adverse effects.

The idea that we need to eat carbohydrates every few hours to keep our energy up is a myth.

Insulin and Carbohydrate Handling

The digestion of a meal containing carbohydrates causes blood sugar (glucose) levels to rise. In response, the pancreas gland secretes insulin into the bloodstream to keep sugar levels from rising too high. The insulin drives the excess sugar out of the blood, into our tissues. Once inside the tissues' cells, the glucose will be used as an immediate energy source or stored for later use. Excessive sugar is stored either as body fat or as glycogen in liver and muscle.

When we digest fats, we see very little direct effect on blood sugar levels. That's because fat contains almost no carbohydrate. In fact, when fats are eaten with high-carbohydrate foods, it tends to slow the rise and peak in blood sugar you'd see if you had eaten the carbohydrates alone.

Ingested protein can and does raise blood sugar, usually to a mild degree. As proteins are digested, our bodies can make sugar (glucose) out of the breakdown products. The healthy pancreas releases some insulin to keep the blood sugar from going too high.

In contrast to fats and proteins, carbohydrates in food cause significant and often dramatic rises in blood sugar. Our pancreas, in turn, secretes higher amounts of insulin to prevent excessive elevation of blood glucose. Carbohydrates are easily digested and converted into blood sugar. The exception is fiber, which is indigestible and passes through us unchanged.

During the course of a day, the pancreas of a healthy person produces an average of 40 to 60 units of insulin. Half of that insulin is secreted in response to meals, the other half is steady state or "basal" insulin. The exact amount of insulin depends quite heavily on the amount and timing of carbohydrates eaten. Dietary protein has much less influence. A pancreas in a healthy person eating a very-low-carbohydrate diet will release substantially less than 50 units of insulin a day.

To summarize thus far: dietary carbohydrates are the major source of blood sugar for most people eating "normally." Carbohydrates are, in turn, the main cause for insulin release by the pancreas, to keep blood sugar levels in a safe, healthy range.

You've learned that insulin's main action is to lower blood sugar by transporting it into the cells of various tissues. But that's not all insulin does. It also 1) impairs breakdown of glycogen into glucose, 2) stimulates glycogen formation, 3) inhibits formation of new glucose molecules by the body, 4) promotes storage of triglycerides in fat cells (i.e., lipogenesis, fat accumulation), 5) promotes formation of fatty acids (triglyceride building blocks) by the liver, 6) inhibits breakdown of stored triglycerides, and 7) supports body protein production.

Insulin actions No.4 and No.5 are particularly problematic if you're trying to get rid of excess body fat. To paraphrase: insulin promotes storage of body fat and impairs breakdown of existing fat tissue. Not good if you want to get rid of excess fat. In that instance, wouldn't it make sense to try to reduce insulin release by the pancreas? You do that by cutting down on easily digestible carbohydrates like sugar-sweetened drinks and refined flours and starches. Or reduce total carbohydrate consumption. Or both.

Now close your book and take out a clean sheet of paper and a pencil for a pop quiz.

Just kidding! Don't sweat it. You won't have to remember all this stuff to be successful with the Advanced Mediterranean Diet.

VITAMINS

I vividly recall a patient of mine, a known alcoholic, who was brought to the emergency room by his wife because he was unable to walk without help. He was fine until a few days earlier when he noticed spells of double vision. I found him also to be confused and cross-eyed. He wasn't drunk. His prompt improvement after an infusion of a specific vitamin into his blood-stream confirmed my suspicion: he had a thiamine deficiency.

Vitamins are organic substances that are vitally necessary in small amounts for normal growth and activity of our bodies. All can be obtained naturally from food. We only need tiny amounts since they are not energy sources or tissue building blocks.

Thus far in nutritional science, 13 vitamins have been identified. They are divided into categories based on whether they dissolve in water or fat/oil.

The water-soluble vitamins are vitamin C, the B vitamins (thiamine (B1), riboflavin (B2), niacin (nicotinic acid), biotin, pantothenic acid, B6 (pyridoxine), folate (folic acid), and B12 (cobalamin).

The fat-soluble vitamins are A, D, E, and K.

Fat-soluble vitamins are stored in our fat tissue and are released to the other tissues as needed over weeks or months. Water-soluble vitamins generally cannot be stored; excess intake is flushed out quickly by the kidneys. The take-home point: we need to eat water-soluble vitamins almost every day.

Vitamin deficiency diseases are uncommon in the developed world, thanks to an abundance of various foods and food fortification with added vitamins (e.g., flour with folate, milk with vitamin D). In fact, disorders of vitamin overdosage may be more common than deficiency. It's a different story in parts of the Third World. Vitamin A deficiency, for example, is a major nutritional problem in the developing world, contributing to childhood blindness and premature death from infections.

Each vitamin has a specific job description in the business of nutritional physiology. Vitamins typically assist the enzymes that govern all the chemical reactions that constitute life. Here's a sampler of vitamin functions:

- assist cell growth and multiplication of cells (B vitamins)
- assist energy production (B vitamins)
- promote nerve growth and protection (B12)
- serve as anti-oxidants that interfere with free radicals, thereby preventing damage to cell structures and alteration of normal cell functions (C, E)
- help with formation of collagen, the major structural protein in connective tissue
- help with formation of thyroid hormone and epinephrine
- promote healthy bones (A, D, K)
- essential to vision (A)

■ help with formation of proteins that are responsible for blood clotting (K).

Lack of a single vitamin can kill you. Until the mid-18th century, sailors on long voyages commonly suffered that fate. Vegetables and fruits deteriorated more rapidly than other food provisions, so they were eaten early in the voyage. Later on, sailors predictably developed easy bruising, bleeding gums, poor wound healing, joint pains, and progressive weakness. Many eventually died from the disease scurvy. Suspecting a nutritional deficiency as the cause, a British physician in 1747 discovered that lime juice prevented the illness. To this day, "limey" is a slang term for a British sailor. Scientists later identified the single vital substance in lime juice as vitamin C.

Although vitamins are individually necessary for life, it is important to know that they work in concert with each other and with the other nutrients. Like the individual musicians in an orchestra, all the vitamins must be present and balanced to produce a beautiful work of art.

Full-blown vitamin deficiencies are rare in developed Western cultures. It is certainly possible, yet difficult to prove, that many people have mild vitamin (and mineral) deficiencies causing fatigue, malaise, weakness, lethargy, dizziness, or other non-specific symptoms. Other causes are usually responsible. But without a doubt, such symptoms sometimes improve when a poor diet is altered to include a greater amount and variety of vitamins and minerals.

Several professional nutrition associations have recommended that healthy, non-pregnant adults not use vitamin supplements ordinarily. There are well-defined important exceptions to the general rule, so you should not stop a supplement recommended by your physician or registered dietitian. Most nutrition professionals recommend you obtain all your vitamins and other nutrients from a variety of whole foods: fruits, vegetables, grains, legumes, nuts, dairy products, fish, meat, poultry, and eggs.

To be absolutely certain you are getting all your necessary vitamins, I recommend you take a multivitamin when you start Ketogenic Mediterranean Diet.

MINERALS

Like the preceding nutrients we have reviewed, minerals are necessary for life. "Organic" nutrients are primarily based on the carbon atom and include fats, proteins, carbohydrates, and vitamins. In contrast, minerals are not based on carbon. They are inorganic elements that can carry an electrical charge when dissolved in water.

Our major minerals, in order of decreasing amounts in the body, are calcium, phosphorus, potassium, sulfur, sodium, chloride, and magnesium. The levels of all the minerals are tightly controlled by the kidneys, gastrointestinal tract, cell walls, hormones, and certain vitamins. Major minerals are most notable for their roles in:

- fluid balance, both inside and outside of cells
- regulation of acid-base balance
- structure of skeleton and teeth
- proper nerve and muscle function.

The average person has 2.5 pounds (1.1 kg) of calcium, 99% of which is in bones and teeth, contributing to structural integrity of the body. Calcium is also essential for blood clotting and function of muscles and nerves.

Phosphorus (1.5 pounds or 0.7 kg) is also a major component of bones and teeth. It is also important in acid-base balance, energy metabolism (e.g., adenosine triphosphate), cell walls (e.g., phospholipids), and in DNA-RNA.

Fluid balance is particularly dependent on sodium, chloride, and potassium.

Magnesium plays important roles in muscle and nerve function, protein production, energy metabolism, and bone mineralization.

Sulfur helps determine the shape of many protein molecules (e.g., insulin) and is a component of some vitamins and amino acids.

Minerals present in much smaller amounts, while still necessary for life, are called trace minerals. All together, our trace minerals might fill a couple thimbles. The most important trace minerals are iron, manganese, copper, iodide, selenium, zinc, fluoride, chromium, molybdenum, arsenic, nickel, silicon, and boron.

We've reviewed basic isolated attributes of water, fats, carbohydrates, proteins, vitamins, and minerals. Now let's tie it all together.

THE BIG PICTURE

Every single bite of food you swallow will be used in one or more of three possible ways:
1. for immediate energy
2. stored as energy (as fat or glycogen)

3. growth, maintenance, or repair of tissues.

While maintenance and repair of tissues are important to all of us, growth is a major issue in children, adolescents, and pregnant women. Proteins are the primary ingredient for growth and tissue maintenance and repair. That's why we eat proteins. They are not major energy-yielding nutrients.

We obtain energy from the chemical bonds between atoms in nutrients. The main energy-yielding nutrients are carbohydrates and fats. Chemical reactions break the bonds between the atoms, releasing the energy stored in the bonds. Much more energy can be released when oxygen is used in energy-producing chemical reactions. We huff and puff during exercise so we can pick up and deliver more oxygen to working muscle cells. Heavy breathing also blows off the carbon dioxide that is a by-product of energy metabolism.

We must have energy to fuel two fundamental life processes: 1) basal metabolism, and 2) physical activity.

BASAL METABOLIC RATE

Basal metabolism refers to all the physiologic processes and chemical reactions that keep us alive in a resting state. These include maintenance of body temperature, breathing, continuous blood production, routine maintenance of healthy tissues, 100,000 heartbeats daily, etc. About 70% of our energy intake is used just for basal metabolism. Basal metabolic rate (BMR) is the rate at which the body uses energy (calories) for life-maintaining activities while lying down in a comfortable room with an empty stomach. These processes may require

1,200 to 1,500 calories per day for an average person, although there is large variability.

While heredity has a significant effect on BMR, a number of other conditions also affect it, and some are under our control. Factors that increase BMR include youth, tall and thin physique, growth (including pregnancy), higher muscle mass, stress, hot or cold environment, and overactive thyroid. Factors that decrease BMR include aging, excess fat tissue, fasting, starvation, malnutrition, and underactive thyroid.

There's no quick, easy, safe way to increase basal metabolic rate. If there were, losing excess weight would be a cinch. We would simply rev up our metabolism and fuel it with the energy stored in fat.

ENERGY EXPENDITURE

In addition to basal metabolism, the other major component of energy expenditure has the potential to convert our excess fat to actual energy. That component is physical activity. In theory, it sounds easy to increase exercise levels and burn off excess fat. In reality, it's difficult and usually doesn't make a major contribution to loss of excess weight.

Why doesn't exercise work better? It's not entirely clear, but a number of issues undoubtedly come into play. Exercise may stimulate appetite and lead to higher food consumption. It may be too hard to stick with a rigorous program. In terms of weight management, it's much easier to just skip the candy bar than to jog on a treadmill for 45 minutes to burn off the calories in the candy.

Muscles move us about by contracting, which requires energy. Heart rate and breathing rate increase above basal rates to supply muscles with oxygen and nutrients, and remove waste byproducts. On average, we use 20 to 30% of our energy on physical activity. An athlete in a vigorous training program may use 60 to 70% of his energy for exercise and only 30 to 40% for basal metabolism.

Physical activity in adulthood tends to decrease an average of 3% per decade, likely contributing to weight gain.

ENERGY PRODUCTION

Food is composed of various atoms bonded together. These bonds contain energy that is released when the bonds are broken by digestive and metabolic processes. The familiar calorie is a measurement of the energy-producing potential contained in food.

Fat is an excellent source of calories, with nine calories per gram. (A gram is about the weight of an aspirin tablet.) Carbohydrate and protein have four calories per gram. Alcohol can also provide energy: seven calories per gram. Most foods are a combination of carbohydrate, protein, fat, vitamins, and minerals. Carbohydrates and fats are our major sources of energy.

Carbohydrates (via glucose) are the best source of immediate energy. Fats are the next best source. We can train our bodies to use fats rather than carbohydrates as the primary energy source. When carbohydrates and fats are not available, the body will use amino acids for energy, even if it has to break down its own proteins to get amino acids for conversion to glucose. Remember that the brain and nerves must have glucose. If proteins are consumed in excess of the body's need for amino acids, they are converted into an immediate energy supply (glucose) or to fat. Excess amino acids cannot be stored for use later. On the other hand, if we don't eat enough protein, our body proteins break down to supply essential amino acids needed more urgently elsewhere in the body. Over time, this leads to muscle wasting.

BALANCED NUTRITON

All the aforementioned chemical reactions require the presence and proper balance of all the various nutrients, including vitamins and minerals. As an example, consider the major blood protein called hemoglobin. Iron is a key component of this large molecule, although it is primarily composed of amino acids derived from protein you eat. Let's say you eat plenty of protein. But if you don't ingest enough iron, you won't be able to make adequate amounts of hemoglobin. You'll be anemic; you won't have enough blood and will feel tired all the time.

ENERGY BALANCE EQUATION

Since you're interested in losing weight, you must never forget that the energy content of everything you eat will either be used as energy within hours, or stored as fat or glycogen.

Nearly all the energy we ingest as food is used within hours to fuel basal metabolism or physical activity. This is true even for grossly obese people. If your weight is stable over time, you are in "energy balance," even if you weigh 350 pounds (159 kg). You're burning up as many calories as you take in. If you've gradually gained 10 pounds (4.5 kg) over the last two years, your energy equation is slightly out of balance: you've eaten more energy than your body needed, and the excess is stored in your adipose tissue. If you wish to lose weight, you must tip the balance in the other direction, converting fat into the energy your body needs. There are only three ways to do this: 1) eat less food, 2) increase your basal metabolic rate, or 3) increase your physical activity.

The living human organism is an incredibly complex system. In terms of fundamental understanding of life, scientists have only scratched the surface. But they've discovered enough details so that you can become and stay healthy for as long as possible. But such knowledge is useless to you unless applied.

KEY POINTS

- Metabolism is the sum of chemical and physical processes necessary for the maintenance of life.
- Good health requires the proper mix of nutrients: water, fat, protein, carbohydrates, vitamins, and minerals.
- Nine of the amino acids we need can be obtained only from proper food choices, so they are essential.
- The two essential fatty acids, linoleic and linolenic, can only be obtained through correct food choices.
- There are no "essential carbohydrates" that we must obtain from food.
- Vitamins are organic substances that are vitally necessary in small amounts for normal growth and activity. Lack of a single vitamin can kill you.

- We must eat water-soluble vitamins frequently since we cannot store them in our bodies as we do fat-soluble vitamins.
- Every single bite of food you swallow will be used in one of three ways: 1) for immediate energy, 2) for growth, maintenance, or repair of tissues, or 3) stored as energy in the form of glycogen or fat.
- The two determinants of our fuel requirements are basal metabolism and physical activity.
- If you wish to lose weight, there are only three possible ways: 1) eat less, 2) increase your basal metabolic rate, or 3) increase your physical activity.

3

I'm Fat. So What?

"I'm sorry, Matt, but we gave the promotion to Carlos," said Matt's boss. "You're a great employee and we don't want to lose you, but we have to do what's best for the company. I'm glad to give you a 3% raise. Thanks for your loyal service."

Matt was a graphic designer for an advertising agency. He had been with the company for four years. The quality of his work couldn't be beat. He was funny and likable. His attendance and timeliness were impeccable. He enjoyed brainstorming with the other designers if they needed help meeting their deadlines, even if he had to stay late. Matt had been awarded "Employee of the Year" after his third year with the agency. He was the "go-to guy" for many of the account executives when they needed fresh ideas.

Carlos, on the other hand, had been with the firm for only two years. The quality of his work was OK, but it was clear he would never set the advertising world on fire. He always clocked out at five o'clock sharp. As might be expected in an advertising firm, image was everything. The company owners and most of the bosses were fitness buffs. Several were known to have had cosmetic surgery. Carlos regaled the bosses and office ladies with his tales of rock climbing and competitive cycling. To top it off, Carlos was a dead ringer for Antonio Banderas.

The promotion involved the agency's first satellite office on the other side of the city. They needed a chief designer who would have creative control and supervise three other designers. The position would have almost doubled Matt's salary. Matt couldn't help but wonder if his weight, 325 pounds (148 kg), was the reason he was passed over. He didn't fit the corporate image of sleek and fit. He recalled the time a year previously his office chair collapsed under him. Everyone heard the commotion and rushed over. Was it his weight, or a defective chair that would have dumped anyone? His co-workers were too kind to speculate out loud. But, even now, Matt felt a rush of anxiety just thinking about the incident.

Matt had always been fat, even in childhood. He didn't know why. His parents were a little over-weight, about like everyone else. He was too heavy in childhood to do well in sports, so he developed other interests and talents. He dated girls occasionally, but even less after he graduated from college. Women didn't seem too interested in him romantically. Many just wanted to be friends.

Matt was sedentary. Given the choice of walking up a flight of stairs or taking the elevator, he always took the lift. He wondered, periodically, if he could slim down by exercising. His friends invited him to participate in their team sports, but he turned them down, fearing that he would drag down the team's performance with his weight and lack of physical fitness. He tried walking outside regularly, even though that was quite difficult after he passed 275 pounds (125 kg). It also bored him to tears. Five months out of the year it was too hot and humid even for walking. Tennis was hard on his ankles. His weight exceeded the limit for a rowing shell. He enjoyed bocce, but couldn't find other players. Golf was too expensive and time-consuming. Miniature golf didn't burn many calories. He was in a bowling league, but realized it wasn't much of a workout. Bicycling gave him a rash "down there."

Recently, Matt had been sleeping poorly at night and was sleepy during the day. He didn't feel well-rested when he woke up in the morning. His housemate noted that Matt snored loudly and tossed and turned all night long, although he seemed to be asleep. He even seemed to stop breathing for brief spells while asleep. Matt figured his sagging mattress was the problem, so he replaced it even though he was only four years into the 10-year warranty. It didn't help. Matt, age 28, came to see me for help with daytime sleepiness.

PSYCHOSOCIAL ASPECTS

Nobody ever says anything good about being overweight, but there are advantages. By putting stress on the bones, obesity keeps them strong and prevents osteoporosis. Fat tissue fills in wrinkles, making the skin look younger. Abundant fat stores serve as insulation, conserving body heat, and allow you to survive longer during periods of starvation. Since

63

many of us currently don't consider excessive weight to be physically attractive, obesity can help you avoid unwanted sexual advances. Physical attractiveness is associated with higher income, but also lower scores on IQ tests and, in women, with being less satisfied with life in middle age. Being overweight and unconcerned about the consequences lets you eat all the delicious food you can get your lips on.

Actually, there is an organization that says good things about being overweight: the National Association to Advance Fat Acceptance. Founded in 1969, NAAFA is "dedicated to protecting the rights and improving the quality of life for fat people. NAAFA works to eliminate discrimination based on body size and provide fat people with the tools for self-empowerment through advocacy, public education, and support."

But there's another side to this coin. Are the advantages of fatness worth the teasing, the loss of mobility, the nagging from relatives and friends, the social isolation? Are they worth the extra wear and tear on furniture and clothing, the embarrassment of not fitting in the seat of an airplane or theater, the feelings of failure and inferiority, the adverse discrimination in social and job settings? I'm neither condoning nor justifying any of these situations; they are simply reality for many obese people. Psychosocial disadvantages reflect primarily the culture in which we find ourselves, and secondarily the people around us.

ECONOMICS

In the United States in 2009, the direct yearly medical cost of being obese was $1,723 (USD) per obese person, according to a report in *Obesity Reviews*. Being merely overweight was a relative bargain at $266. These numbers translated into $114 billion yearly, or five to 10% of total healthcare spending. A large majority of that money is spent on diabetes and cardiovascular disease associated with obesity.

Overweight people spend at least $60 billion (USD) yearly in the United States on various weight-loss efforts.

HEALTH CONSEQUENCES

OVERALL ILLNESS AND DEATH

The numerous obesity-related illnesses are more common and severe the longer obesity has been present. And as might be expected, the fatter, the riskier. A typical high-risk person would be a 45-year-old who has weighed 260 pounds (118 kg) since the age of 20. Associated illnesses may simply cause pain (e.g., gallstones, arthritis), or contribute to premature death (e.g., heart attacks, high blood pressure).

Looking at all overweight and obese people as a group, the death rate is probably only mildly higher than would be expected otherwise. But the mortality rate gradually starts rising at a body mass index (BMI) of 30 (e.g., a 5-foot, 4-inch (163 cm) person weighing 174 pounds (79 kg) or a 5-foot, 10-inch (178 cm) person weighing 207 pounds or 94 kg). A major increase in medical complications, and much of the premature deaths, occurs in those who have a body mass index over 40 (e.g., a 5-foot, 4-inch (163 cm) person weighing 240 pounds (109 kg) or a 5-foot, 10-inch (178 cm) person weighing 310 pounds or 141 kg).

You can find your own body mass index if you know your weight and height by using an online calculator such as the one at http://advancedmediterraneandiet.com/bmicalcula tor.html

A 25-year-old morbidly obese man (e.g., 5-foot, 10-inch (178 cm) tall, 280 pounds or 127 kg)) will die 12 years sooner than otherwise expected, on average.

Obesity is involved in five of the top 10 causes of death in the United States. It's quite difficult to calculate how many U.S. deaths are directly attributable to obesity; estimates range from 112,000 to 414,000 per year.

If we look only at older Americans, over 65–75 years old, the condition of being overweight, but not obese, seems to prolong life on average. Longest life spans are seen in older Americans with a body mass index between 25 and 30.

The medical complications of excessive adiposity are somewhat related to distribution of that fat on the body. The two classic distribution patterns are gynoid and android. You can have either pattern whether you are a man or a woman, although your particular pattern is hereditary.

The gynoid pattern is also referred to as lower body, peripheral, or pear-shaped; fat is concentrated on the thighs, buttocks, hips, and lower half of the abdomen.

The android pattern is also called male-type, upper body, abdominal, central, visceral, or apple-shaped; fat is concentrated in the neck, cheeks, shoulders, and abdomen. Distribution of fat in an android or apple-shaped pattern in particular is associated with increased risk of strokes, diabetes, coronary artery disease, high blood pressure, certain cancers, and earlier death.

HIGH BLOOD PRESSURE

At least one-third of all cases of hypertension (high blood pressure) are caused by obesity. Every 20 pounds (9 kg) of excess fat causes a two to three point rise in blood pressure..

DIABETES MELLITUS

There are two types of diabetes mellitus. Type 1 usually starts in childhood and is fatal unless treated with insulin injections. Type 2, or adult-onset diabetes, is much more common and may be managed with diet alone, weight reduction, oral medications, and sometimes insulin. Average age at the time of diagnosis is around 50. Eighty to 90% of all type 2 diabetics are overweight.

The U.S. Centers for Disease Control and Prevention predicts that one of every three Americans born in 2000 will develop diabetes, mostly type 2.

Diabetes is easily diagnosed by finding elevated amounts of sugar (glucose) in the blood. It occurs in 11% of the adults in the United States. That's 26 million cases. In the over-65 crowd, almost one in every three has diabetes (nearly all type 2).

The high sugar levels alone can cause symptoms such as frequent urination and unusual thirst. But diabetes is clearly more complicated than simple "high sugar." Diabetes can impair circulation, nerve and kidney function, and eyesight. Although most diabetics never become blind, diabetes is a leading cause of blindness.

Having diabetes at age 50 more than doubles the risk of developing cardiovascular disease for both women and men.

Compared to those without diabetes, having both cardiovascular disease and diabetes at age 50 approximately doubles the risk of dying, regardless of sex.

Compared to those without diabetes, women and men with diabetes at age 50 die 7 or 8 years earlier, on average.

Clearly, you want to avoid diabetes if you can. A key way to improve your odds is to achieve and maintain a healthy body weight.

PREDIABETES

Prediabetes is defined as 1) having fasting blood sugar between 100 and 125 mg/dl (5.6–6.9 mmol/l), or 2) having blood sugar level of 140–199 mg/dl (7.8–11.1 mmol/l) two hours after drinking 75 grams of glucose.

Overweight and obesity increase your odds of becoming prediabetic. The Centers for Disease Control in 2011 determined that 79 million Americans have prediabetes, including one in three of all adults and half of all those over 65.

Prediabetes is a strong risk factor for development of full-blown diabetes. It's also associated with increased risk for cardiovascular disease such as heart attack and stroke. One of every four adults with prediabetes develops diabetes over the next four years. The progression can often be prevented by lifestyle modifications such as dietary changes, moderate-intensity exercise, and modest weight loss.

GALLSTONES

Gallstones are three or four times more common in the obese. Successful weight loss itself seems to increase the short-term risk of symptomatic gallstones.

CORONARY ARTERY DISEASE

Also known as coronary heart disease, coronary artery disease refers to complications caused by the build-up of plaque in the arteries providing the heart muscle with oxygen and nutrients. The plaque is composed of fats, cholesterol, cells, and debris. The general term for this gradual artery-blocking disease process is atherosclerosis, and it often occurs elsewhere in the body in addition to the heart.

Not uncommonly, the first sign of the problem is sudden death. More fortunate souls may just have a heart attack (aka myocardial infarction, with a 10–25% chance of dying), weakness of the heart muscle (congestive heart failure), or a heart rhythm disturbance.

In overweight people, the risk of developing coronary artery disease is directly related to the degree of fatness, starting at just 10% overweight.

The risk of heart and vascular disease is more closely associated with distribution of excess fat than

69

KMD

with degree of obesity as measured by overall weight or body mass index. Waist-hip ratio (WHR) is a measure of abdominal or central obesity, the type of fat distribution associated with coronary artery disease. This is the android pattern discussed earlier. To determine your waist-hip ratio:

1. While standing, relax your stomach—don't pull it in. Measure around your waist midway between the bottom of the rib cage and the top of your pelvis bone. Usually this is at the level of your belly button, or an inch higher. Don't go above the rib cage. Keep the measuring tape horizontal to the ground and don't compress your skin.
2. Measure around your hips at the widest part of your buttocks. Keep the tape horizontal to the ground and don't compress your skin.
3. Divide the waist by the hip measurement. The result is your waist-hip ratio.

For example, if your waist is 44 inches (112 cm) and hips are 48 inches (122 cm): 44 divided by 48 is 0.92, which is your waist-hip ratio.

Please take the time now to measure and note in your personal records your waist size, hip size, and calculated waist-hip ratio.

Scientists have not yet determined the ideal WHR, but it is probably around 0.85 or less for women, and 0.95 or less for men. Ratios above 1.0 are clearly associated with risk of cardiovascular disease such as heart attacks. The higher the ratio, the higher the risk. Compared with body mass index, WHR is a much stronger predictor of coronary artery disease.

LIPIDS

Obesity tends to elevate total and LDL cholesterol, while lowering HDL cholesterol. LDL is the "bad cholesterol" and HDL is the good. These lipid changes tend to promote atherosclerosis, including coronary artery disease. Furthermore, obesity is associated with high triglycerides, which can cause painful inflammation of the pancreas and may also play a role in atherosclerosis.

CANCER

The incidence of cancer is clearly increased in people who are 40% or more over ideal weight. Men are prone to prostate and colorectal cancers. Women get cancer of the endometrium (uterus), gallbladder, cervix, ovary, and breast. Overweight and obesity are linked to increased risk of kidney cancer and esophageal adenocarcinoma. According to the American Cancer Society, overweight and obesity contribute to 14 to 20 percent of all cancer-related deaths in the United States. Over 500,000 people die from cancer each year in the United States.

RESPIRATORY PROBLEMS

In extremely overweight people, the chest wall and upper airway tissues are so thick and heavy that breathing is impaired. This results in low blood oxygen levels, brief periods during sleep in which breathing stops entirely (obstructive sleep apnea), and daytime sleepiness. My patient, Matt, from the start of this chapter, had sleep apnea.

In contrast, the shortness of breath during exertion experienced by most overweight people is just an indicator of low physical fitness or a reflection of the heavy load they haul.

MISCELLANEOUS CONSEQUENCES

A number of other medical conditions are caused by or associated with obesity:

- Strokes
- Arthritis (especially in the knees)
- Low back pain
- Gout
- Varicose veins
- Hemorrhoids
- Blood clots in the leg veins and lungs
- Complications after surgery, such as wound infection, breathing problems, blood clots, poor wound healing
- Complications during pregnancy, such as toxemia, hypertension, diabetes, prolonged labor, greater need for C-section
- Fat build-up in the liver (hepatic steatosis)
- Delayed or missed diagnosis due to difficult physical examination or weight exceeding the limit of diagnostic equipment
- Asthma
- Menstrual irregularities and decreased fertility
- Low sperm counts and testosterone levels in men

THE GOOD NEWS

Most of the medical consequences of obesity can be significantly improved by losing only 5 to 10% of your weight, sustained over time. This modest weight loss will certainly improve most cases of hypertension, diabetes, and adverse lipids. You don't have to look like a fashion model or a sexy leading man to reap the benefits of long-term weight management.

In fact, you can start very soon to take action that will eliminate or ameliorate ALL of the psychosocial, economic, and medical consequences of overweight. The process has already begun. We have just a little more groundwork to lay before getting down to the nuts and bolts.

KEY POINTS

- Duration and degree of obesity are directly-related to the most serious health consequences of obesity: diabetes, coronary artery disease, strokes, certain cancers, and premature death.
- Apple-shaped obese people suffer more severe medical complications than do pear-shaped.
- Most of the medical consequences of obesity can be significantly improved by losing only 5 to 10% of initial body weight.

I do not like broccoli. And I haven't liked it since I
was a little kid and my mother made me eat it. And
I'm President of the United States and I'm not going
to eat any more broccoli.
— George H.W. Bush, 1990

And you will know the truth, and the truth will
make you free.
— John 8:32

4
A Philosophy of Weight Loss

"**A**re you sure you need that dessert?" asked Amanda's husband. His not-so-subtle references to her excess weight were starting to grate on Amanda's nerves. She didn't need reminders that she was 25 to 30 pounds (11 to 14 kg) overweight. 42-year-old Amanda—5-feet, 6-inches (168 cm) tall—knew she weighed 165 pounds (75 kg).

Amanda and Jim met 13 years earlier. After a year and a half of dating, they married. It was the second marriage for both. Jim retired from the military after 20 years of service and worked as a sheriff's deputy. Amanda was an elementary teacher. She had no children of her own because of medical problems earlier in life. Jim was a good provider. He had a great sense of humor and was a God-fearing man who attended church with her. He'd send her flowers "just because." Jim liked his in-laws. He kept

the yard in tip-top shape and the home in good repair. He was faithful to Amanda for the 11 years of
their marriage. Not uncommonly for ex-military
men, Jim could be a bit of a control freak. Amanda
loved Jim anyway, and felt he loved her back. He
said so. The marriage had hit a few rough patches,
but the couple had worked through them successfully.

Amanda loved the outdoors. She was an avid hiker
and an officer in a hiking club. Two or three week-
ends a month, she would take a four- to eight-mile
strenuous hike either with the club or other friends.
She'd strap on a 15-pound (7 kg) backpack, including camera gear for her nature photography hobby.
Four days a week she'd go for a three-mile walk
with her black Labrador retriever in her neighbor-
hood. Her Lab would often tag along on her hikes
carrying a first-aid kit and his own water in a dog
backpack.

Amanda considered herself 15 pounds (7 kg) overweight when they married. She was 150 pounds (68
kg) at the time. Jim understood he wasn't marrying
a Victoria's Secret model. She gained 10 or 15
pounds (4.5 to 7 kg) over the next five years, but
had held steady since then. She's attractive, and
she knows it. When she's wearing high heels and
dark clothing, the extra weight disappears. Amanda
eats healthy and enjoys her food. If not for Jim's
comments, she'd be comfortable with her current
165 pounds (75 kg). She felt good. Several of the 20-
somethings in the hiking club had trouble keeping
up with her. She doesn't plan on entering the Mrs.
America pageant. Everybody gains a little weight as
they get older, don't they? None of her friends are at
their high school weights. Few are even close.

Nevertheless, over the last couple years Jim had been increasingly critical of her weight. He could stand to lose 40 pounds (18 kg) himself. Their sex life was less active now and Amanda wasn't sure if it was related to her weight, Jim's age (47), or something else entirely. She'd catch his eyes wandering to other women more than usual. He freely shared his idea of feminine perfection with Amanda and her friends: Megan Fox. By the same token, Jim was no Brad Pitt, either. Sure, Amanda wouldn't mind being 135 pounds (61 kg) again, as thin as she was at 25. She wondered if there was an easy, painless way to get there. She wasn't excited about the sacrifices she figured were necessary to lose 30 pounds (14 kg). She'd made some half-hearted attempts at losing weight through calorie-restricted diets, without lasting success. After two or three weeks of deprivation, she couldn't stand the gnawing, unrelenting hunger. She had let Jim know many times that his derogatory weight-related comments cut her to the bone. They quarreled; he apologized. But the hurtful comments began again too soon.

Amanda and Jim's repetitive bickering about her weight started to strain their marriage. In the final analysis, she loved Jim and thought it would just be silly for her weight to jeopardize her marriage. She decided to lose 30 pounds (14 kg) and put an end to his carping. She came to see me for weight-loss pills.

THE ENERGY BALANCE EQUATION

Your fat stores are determined by the number of calories you eat minus the calories you expend ("burn") in physical activities and resting metabolism. This is the energy balance equation introduced earlier.

Obesity results from an imbalance between calorie intake and calorie expenditure. The degree of this imbalance may be quite small. Over the course of a year, all other things being equal, you'll gain three and a half pounds (1.6 kg) of fat just by adding a teaspoon (5 ml) of butter to your dinner roll every day.

I have no doubt that the energy balance equation applies to you. People who swear they can't lose weight on extreme low-calorie diets have been locked up (with consent) in university medical center metabolic wards with access to food strictly controlled by staff. On appropriate calorie-restricted diets, everyone loses weight. When an exercise program is added, they lose more weight.

The only way to lose weight is to cut down on the calories you take in, increase your physical activity, or do both. Although the exercise portion of the equation is somewhat optional, you must reduce food intake to lose a significant amount of weight.

GRAND UNIFICATION THEORY

In the Introduction, I told you about Gary Taubes' "carbohydrate/insulin theory of obesity." To recap: The main hormone in charge of fat storage is insulin; it works to make us fatter, building fat tissue. If you've got too much fat, you must have too much insulin action. And what drives insulin secretion from your pancreas? Dietary carbohydrates, especially refined carbs such as sugars, flour, cereal grains, and starchy vegetables (e.g., corn, beans, rice, potatoes). These are the "fattening carbs." Dozens of enzymes and hormones are at play either depositing fat into tissue, or mobilizing the fat to be used as energy. It's an active process going on continuously. Any regulatory derangement that favors fat accumulation will *cause* gluttony (overeating) or sloth (inactivity).

I think both the energy balance equation and carbohydrate/insulin theory have validity and practical application for weight management. Several studies of very-low-carbohydrate dieting show that successful dieters have reduced their calorie consumption from baseline, which supports the energy balance equation theory. By the same token, many people have lost weight on high-carbohydrate diets by reducing calories from pre-diet levels. For at least a few people, exercise does indeed accelerate the rate of weight loss. In favor of the carbohydrate/insulin theory are numerous studies finding greater degrees of weight loss, with less hunger and better compliance, on very-low-carbohydrate diets.

Undoubtedly, we all have metabolisms that differ from others because of heredity and other factors. Calorie-restricted dieting may work better for one metabolic type, whereas very-low-carbohydrate, eat-all-you-want dieting works better for another. For those who prefer a calorie-restricted diet, I recommend *The Advanced Mediterranean Diet* (2nd edition).

Both dieter types, however, need to incorporate willpower, commitment, knowledge, motivation, discipline, and social support. Success depends on them.

WILLPOWER AND FREE WILL

Are you able to reduce calorie intake and increase your physical activity level? Can you break your sugar-sweetened beverage habit? Will you turn down the cake and ice cream at the office party?

It boils down to whether we have free will. Free will is the power, attributed especially to humans, of making free choices that are unconstrained by external circumstances or by an agency such as divine will. Will is the mental faculty by which one chooses or decides upon a course of action; volition. Willpower is the strength of will to carry out one's decisions, wishes, or plans.

If we don't have free will, you're wasting time with this book; nothing will get your weight problem under control. Even liposuction and weight-reduction stomach surgery will fail in time if you are fated to be fat. I believe we have free will. I've seen hundreds of my patients lose weight and keep it under control. I didn't do it for them. No other person, pill, or agency did it for them. They didn't achieve success by being passive victims of external circumstances. They did it by exercising their free will.

COMMITMENT

Your success in weight loss and long-term management are dependent on commitment and willpower. In most cases, if not all, a change in lifestyle will be necessary. This isn't easy. Your commitment and willpower will be fortified by knowledge, motivation, discipline, and social support.

KNOWLEDGE

You have learned how your body needs various nutrients, how it stores excess energy intake as fat, how it can convert fat to energy as needed for physical activity and metabolism. You know the adverse health consequences of excess fat and soon will learn about the beneficial effects of exercise. This knowledge will support your commitment and will-power.

MOTIVATION

Immediate, short-term motivation to lose weight may stem from an upcoming high school reunion, swimsuit season, or a wedding. You want to look your best. Maybe you want to attract a mate or keep one interested. Perhaps a boyfriend, co-worker, or relative said something mean about your weight. These motivators may work, but only temporarily. Basing a lifestyle change on them is like building on shifting sands. You need a firmer foundation for a lasting structure. Proper long-term motivation may grow from:

- the discovery that you feel great and have more energy when you're lighter and eating sensibly
- the sense of accomplishment from steady progress
- the acknowledgment that you have free will and are responsible for your weight and many aspects of your health
- the inspiration from seeing others take charge of their lives successfully
- the admission that you have some guilt and shame about being fat, and that you like yourself more when you're not fat
- the awareness of obesity-related health problems and their improvement with even modest weight loss

Appropriate motivation will support your commitment and willpower.

DISCIPLINE

You already have a number of good habits that support your health and make your life more enjoyable, productive, and efficient. For example, you brush your teeth and bathe regularly, put away clean clothes in particular spots, pay bills on time, get up and go to work every day, wear your seat belt, put your keys or purse in one place when you get home, balance your checkbook periodically. At one point, these habits took much more effort than they do now. But you decided they were the right thing to do, made them a priority, practiced them at first, made a conscious effort to perform them on schedule, and repeated them over time.

All this required discipline. That's how good habits become part of your lifestyle, part of you. Over time, your habits require much less effort and hardly any thought. You just do it. Your decision to lose fat permanently means that you must establish some new habits, such as reasonable food restriction and regular exercise. You've already demonstrated that you have self-discipline. The application of that discipline to new behaviors will support your commitment and willpower.

SOCIAL SUPPORT

Success at any major endeavor is easier when you have a supportive social system. Your starring role in a weight-loss program may win an Academy Award if you have a strong cast of supporting actors. Your mate, friends, co-workers, and relatives may help or hinder you. It will help if they:
- give you encouragement instead of criticism
- don't tempt you with taboo foods

- show respect for your commitment and will-power
- give you time to exercise
- go on a diet or exercise with you, if they're overweight or need exercise
- understand why there are no longer certain foods in the house
- appreciate the nutritious, sensible foods that are now in the house
- forgive and understand when you occasionally backslide
- gently remind you of your commitment when needed
- reward you with compliments as you make progress
- don't compare your physique unfavorably with supermodels or surgically-sculpted bodies
- don't get jealous when you lose weight and are more attractive and energetic.

Your social support system can make or break your commitment and willpower. Ask them to help you.

DIET FAILURE

Nearly everyone can lose weight on nearly any type of popular diet. Diets do work. The problem is that most people quickly regain the fat they lost. The cause usually is a breakdown of motivation, discipline, commitment, willpower, or social support, superimposed on an inadequate knowledge base. In short, people go back to their old ways.

Let me be clear: many diets deserve to fail because they're unsafe and unsustainable from a physiological viewpoint.

Let's dig further into why even reasonable diets fail so often in both the short and long run. And why are you even overweight in the first place?

OVERVIEW

In chapter one, we looked at the the usual causes of overweight and obesity: energy imbalance, fattening carbohydrates (and insulin), physical inactivity, heredity, ancestry, and the thrifty gene hypothesis. (I'll not review here the rare endocrine and central nervous system illnesses that cause obesity.)

We've inherited a biological system designed to store excess energy as fat during times of abundance. The "problem" is that we now live in times of perpetual feast, not famine. Cheap food surrounds us and marketers shower us with titillating ads. In our current obesigenic environment, overweight is the natural condition of humankind.

PSYCHOLOGY

So why isn't everybody fat? It's because of constraints on our behavior that counteract natural tendencies. Nature tells us to eat now and eat well, for tomorrow will bring famine. So get prepared. Nature tells us to kick back and relax while we can, saving our energy for when we really need it. Like for a sprint across the savanna with a brushfire or saber-toothed tiger at our heels! For most of us who are not overweight, it is behavioral constraints that keep us from eating too much, or keep us physically active.

Potential reasons to constrain our eating behavior include fear of negative consequences like bad health outcomes, job discrimination, and poorer prospects of finding and keeping a mate. Use the fear constructively to help you lose weight and get healthier.

Alternatively, we may constrain our eating behavior based on our values or standards. To various degrees, most of us place value in achievement, productivity, discipline, knowledge, willpower, self-improvement, commitment, temperance, hygiene, and self-respect. When we fail to live up to the standards, guilt and shame lead us back to the right path. The potential for guilt and shame inhibits us, i.e., constrains our behavior. On a more positive note, the exhilaration of meeting the standards is its own reward, and diverts our attention from less lofty behavior. These values keep many people from overeating and get them off the couch for exercise when they'd rather watch TV.

EMOTIONAL EATING AND PSYCHIATRIC PROBLEMS

A few overweight people have psychological problems that interfere with weight management. You may be one of them. Depression, anxiety, and other psychological disturbances can be so overwhelming as to block your ability to act on the information presented here. When you're sad, disappointed, angry, discouraged, overworked or stressed out, eating some ice cream, chocolate, cookies, or potato chips provides an immediate emotional boost and short-lived pleasure. Your subconscious remembers that boost. The next time you're upset, you eat. That's food therapy for emotional distress. But it's not the best therapy over the long haul.

Frequent binge eating is probably emotional. A binge is characterized by 1) eating an unusually large amount (1,500 to 20,000 calories) in an hour or two, of typically calorie-dense or "forbidden" foods, 2) a sense of lack of control over eating during the episode, and 3) feelings of disgust, depression, or guilt after overeating. The related disorder, bulimia nervosa, involves recurrent binge eating followed by inappropriate behavior to prevent weight gain, such as laxative abuse, self-induced vomiting, diuretic use, fasting, or excessive exercise.

Instead of reaching for food, many people find emotional relief through other avenues, such as reading, music, volunteer work, exercise, socializing, hobbies, and psychotherapy, to name a few. Careful self-examination may reveal if you're eating to satisfy emotional rather than physiological needs. If you have any doubt, or need help with emotional distress, consult a psychologist, psychiatrist, or trusted religious adviser. Awareness of the problem is half the solution.

Shedding pounds doesn't mean you'll shed job and relationship problems. If you thought losing 50–100 pounds (23–45 kg) would make your life magically better and all problems disappear, don't let the stress of disillusionment precipitate a weight regain. Your life *is* better. Keep slugging away at the problem areas and you'll make progress. It's OK to ask for help.

DIET FAILURE IN TAUBES' MODEL OF OBESITY

In Gary Taubes' model, excessive carbohydrate consumption leads to excessive insulin action, which builds fat tissue. If you fail to lose weight, or regain lost weight, you're simply eating too many carbohydrates. The particularly fattening carbs are sugars and refined starches.

THE LUCKY FEW

Sure, you see people who eat all and anything they want yet don't gain weight. And they're not exercise fanatics. These lucky dogs tend to be either very physically active people, heavy smokers, or active adolescents and young adults with inherently high metabolic rates. After age 30 many of them will start developing "middle-age spread" as metabolism slows and activity levels drop. Nevertheless, it appears that one or two out of every 10 adults need not concern themselves with calories, fat grams, or counting carbohydrates: they will stay slender. Some of them have to push themselves to eat! But you and I need constraints on behavior to keep our weight under control. We're in good company. Just look around!

By the way, when the next prolonged famine hits, you'll outlive that skinny guy if you're carrying some extra fat weight.

WEIGHT GOALS

Deciding how much weight you should lose isn't as simple as it seems at first blush. I rarely have to tell a patient she's overweight. She knows it and has an intuitive sense of whether it's mild, moderate, or severe in degree. She's much less clear about how much weight she should lose.

Several weight standards are in common usage:
   1) Body Mass Index
   2) Aesthetic Ideal Weights
   3) Realistic Weights

BODY MASS INDEX

Body Mass Index (BMI) is your weight in kilograms divided by your height in meters squared (kg/m²). A pound equals 454 kilograms. An inch equals 2.54 centimeters. There are 100 centimeters in one meter. Thus, a 5-foot, 4-inch woman (1.63 meters) weighing 200 pounds (91 kilograms) has a BMI of 34.2. Perhaps you're starting to understand why this weight standard isn't too popular yet.

To learn your own BMI but skip the math, use an online calculator such as this one:
http://advancedmediterraneandiet.com/bmicalculator.html

From a health standpoint, BMIs between 18.5 and 24.9 are the best for people under 65–75 years old. About a third of the United States adult population is at this healthy weight. If your BMI is under 25, any excess fat you carry is unlikely to affect your health and longevity; your efforts to lose weight would be purely cosmetic.

To see if your BMI is in the healthy range of 18.5 to 24.9, find your height in the table below, then look to the healthy weight ranges to the right.

Table of Healthy Weight Ranges Based On Body Mass Index: 18.5 to 24.9

Height (without shoes)	Weight in lb (w/o clothes)	Weight in kg (w/o clothes)
5'0" or 152 cm	95 - 128	43.0 - 58.0
5'1" or 155 cm	98 - 132	44.4 - 59.8
5'2" or 157 cm	101 - 137	45.8 - 62.1
5'3" or 160 cm	105 - 141	47.6 - 63.9
5'4" or 163 cm	108 - 146	48.9 - 66.2

5'5" or 165 mc	111 - 150	50.3 - 68.0
5'6" or 168 cm	115 - 155	52.0 - 70.3
5'7" or 170 cm	118 - 160	53.5 - 72.5
5'8" or 173 cm	122 - 164	55.3 - 74.3
5'9" or 175 cm	125 - 169	51.7 - 76.6
5'10" or 178 cm	129 - 174	58.5 - 78.9
5'11" or 180 cm	133 - 179	60.3 - 81.8
6'0" or 183 cm	137 - 184	62.1 - 83.4
6'1" or 185 cm	140 - 189	63.5 - 85.7
6'2" or 188 cm	144 - 195	65.3 - 88.4
6'3" or 191 cm	148 - 200	67.1 - 90.7
6'4" or 193 cm	152 - 205	68.9 - 92.9

BMIs between 25 and 29.9 designate "overweight." A BMI of 30 or higher defines "obesity" and indicates high risk for poor health. At BMI of 35 and above, the risk of death and disease increases sharply.

The BMI concept is helpful to researchers and obesity clinicians, even thought it's not a prefect gauge of weight-related illness risk.

AESTHETIC IDEAL WEIGHT

Aesthetic Ideal Weights are somewhat personal, although clearly influenced by culture. You know without much thought at what weight you look your best. Whether others agree with you, and whether you could realistically hope to reach that weight, are entirely different matters.

If your personal Aesthetic Ideal Weight matches the Hollywood hunk or sex kitten actress du jour, prepare for failure. Thespians and models want to be thin because the camera puts weight on them. Many of our beloved photogenic celebrities workout three hours daily with a personal trainer. And on top of that, many also visit plastic surgeons. I suggest you pull your head out of the stars, come back to earth, find a friend with your type of body frame and height who looks "normal" to you. What does he or she weigh? Now you've got something to shoot for. I also suggest validation of your Aesthetic Ideal Weight by a trusted adviser.

REALISTIC WEIGHTS

A Realistic Weight goal is one that you have a reasonable expectation of achieving, accompanied by significant psychological or medical benefits. This standard is flexible. There's no weight chart to consult since your potential psychological or medical benefits are unique. These weights tend to be higher than the other benchmarks thus far reviewed.

Remember, many of the illnesses caused or aggravated by obesity are improved significantly by loss of only 5 or 10% of body weight, regardless of final weight or body mass index.

The Realistic Weight concept accepts that you can feel better, look better, and have fewer medical problems while falling far short of the healthy BMI of 18.5 to 24.9.

It's not realistic to expect a 40-year-old mother of three to look like a 17-year-old with no kids. It's clearly not impossible, but you just don't see it very often. Nor is there a need for it. The Realistic Weight concept also accounts for personal history and recognizes a point of diminishing returns, i.e., increasing effort with decreasing payoff.

For example, consider a diabetic with high blood pressure, 5-foot, 10-inches tall (178 cm), weighing

300 pounds (136 kg) for the last 20 years. His BMI is 44.5. He loses weight down to 215 pounds (98 kg), feels great, looks much better, cured his diabetes, and was able to stop one of his blood pressure medicines with his doctor's blessing. His BMI is now 31. But his body is starting to resist further weight loss. It's an increasing struggle for him, and he's not very close to his "ideal" healthy weight of 173 pounds or 79 kg (BMI 24.9). At 215 pounds (98 kg) he has gained most of the health and psychological benefits of weight loss, probably adding years to his life. 215 pounds (98 kg) isn't perfect, but it's good. He's lost 85 pounds (39 kg) of fat, which is a major accomplishment. Rejoice and be happy! For many people, the Realistic Weight concept is helpful and valid, and prevents the discouragement felt when performance falls short of ideal. Let's not allow the perfect to be the enemy of the good.

DOC, HOW MUCH WEIGHT SHOULD I LOSE?

As a medical man, I endorse the healthy BMI concept (BMI 18.5 to 24.9) while realizing you may have aesthetic reasons to shoot for the lower end of the range. If you have weight-related health issues, aim for a BMI of 18.5-24.9, with 25 to 30 as your fallback position. If you're over 65, consider a goal BMI between 25 and 30. Elderly Americans tend to live longest at BMIs of 25 to 30, although disability in that age group is lowest at a BMI of 24.

Please take the time now to measure and note in your personal records today's date and your:

Weight
Height
Waist size
Hip size

Waist-hip ratio
Current BMI
Weight goal

ARE YOU SURE YOU WANT TO LOSE WEIGHT?

The weight-loss program I recommend to you is not easy. You won't lose eight pounds (3.6 kg) of fat the first week and 20 pounds (9 kg) the first month. Progress is slow. It will require major lifestyle and attitude changes on your part, perhaps even by your household members. I realize I may scare you away and lose book sales by admitting all this, but it's the truth. Look elsewhere if you want a fast, easy solution—you'll be back. Successfully losing weight and keeping it off by any method is hard.

So why follow the Ketogenic Mediterranean Diet? It respects your individuality. It's relatively inexpensive. It will improve your health and sense of well-being. It's realistic and relatively convenient. It works. The program I propose to you has worked for my patients. Sure, it's tough. But they did it. You can do it, too.

Now back to Amanda's story, from the beginning of this chapter. Her husband was hounding her to lose weight, to look more like Megan Fox. All other things being equal, she was satisfied with her weight at 165 pounds (75 kg). But his nagging and their subsequent quarrelling were straining their marriage. She came to me for weight-loss pills to help her lose 30 pounds (14 kg). I found Amanda to be in perfect health, except her body mass index was mildly above the healthy range of 18.5 to 24.9. Hers was 26.7. Her strenuous hiking demonstrated the vigor of her cardiovascular, pulmonary, and musculoskeletal systems. All of her laboratory studies were normal, including cholesterol levels, trig-lycerides, blood sugar, and thyroid. Nearly all of her blood relatives lived to be over 85 and were robust until the end, eventually dying of "old age." I expected Amanda's health and longevity to follow the path of her relatives. I saw no medical reason for Amanda to lose weight. Any weight loss would be purely cosmetic.

I pointed out to Amanda that her net weight gain over her 11 years of marriage was only 15 pounds (7 kg), and it seemed to me Jim was blowing it all out of proportion. She had a bigger problem than 15 pounds (7 kg) of fat. I strongly suspected that the nagging and bickering were about something other than her weight. If so, losing the weight would not get to the heart of the matter, and the strain in the marriage would persist. Amanda didn't need weight-loss pills, or weight loss. I recommended they see their pastor for marital counseling. I knew the pastor had a good reputation for couples therapy, and he would be in a position to drill down to, and deal with, the core issues. Amanda and Jim needed talk therapy, not pill therapy. It turns out my hunch was correct: Jim had issues he needed to address. He did so, and the marriage improved. Among other things, the pastor recommended they spend more time together, so Jim started hiking with her regularly. He lost 20 pounds (9 kg) over the next year.

KEY POINTS

- We tend to eat more and exercise less than we realize.
- Successful weight management requires commitment, knowledge, motivation, social support, discipline, and willpower.

- From now on, you'll have to constrain your natural eating inclinations.
- A Realistic Weight goal is one that you have a reasonable expectation of achieving, accompanied by significant psychological or medical benefits. Oftentimes this is good enough.
- The healthy Body Mass Index range is 18.5 to 24.9.
- If you have medical problems caused or aggravated by obesity, aim for a Body Mass Index under 25. If that's not possible, be proud and happy with reduction to a BMI of 25 to 30, or with loss of 5 to 10% of your initial weight.

4
Two Diets: Moderate and Radical

Historically, respected and balanced weight-loss programs followed an established formula based on the energy balance equation. You know the drill: eat less, exercise more. This is calorie-restricted eating. Followers make moderate changes to their eating habits.

Alternatively, a radical approach to weight management is to drastically reduce consumption of fattening carbohydrates. Scientific evidence in favor of this approach has been accumulating over the last decade. This chapter explores the pros and cons of each method.

CALORIE-RESTRICTED DIETING

Reduced-calorie eating has a number of appeals. The dieter can often stick with familiar foods, which increases compliance with the program. Changes in diet can be made gradually, which appeals to many folks. A well-balanced eating plan is very safe from a health standpoint, with little risk of precipitating hair loss, lack of energy, low blood sugar, rashes, headaches, fatigue, easy bruising, etc.

Clearly, I'm not talking about starvation diets or very-low-calorie diets here. Cutting daily calorie consumption below 1,200 for most women or below 1,500 for most men is unsustainable and possibly dangerous.

Calorie-restricted diets with or without an exercise component do indeed work, if followed. Sure, results may only be temporary, but that's an issue for all diets.

A major focus of mine for the last 15 years has been to educate my patients sufficiently that they'll stick with such a program and maintain their success long-term. The sum total of my educational efforts is *The Advanced Mediterranean Diet* (2nd edition). It's a moderate, reduced-calorie, balanced diet with an exercise component. It's worked well for many folks. For details, see
http://AdvancedMediterraneanDiet.com

But it doesn't work for everybody. No single diet will. Advanced Mediterranean Diet non-responders and backsliders often do better with my radical Ketogenic Mediterranean Diet.

Here's a thumbnail sketch of the Advanced Mediterranean Diet. Based on your weight and sex, you're assigned a caloric intake level. Then I teach you how to approximate the traditional, healthy Mediterranean diet by eating specified amounts of whole grains, vegetables, fruits, fats, diary products, and high-protein foods. Huge amount of variety in terms of foods and how to prepare them. I think it's a great program and have followed it myself.

This reduced-calorie approach to weight loss, coupled with exercise, is traditional and popular with dietitians and physicians.

However, the Advanced Mediterranean Diet is not without criticism from some quarters. One drawback is that you have to measure food and keep a fairly detailed record of consumption. If you've eaten your allocation of food for the day and you're still hungry, you can't do much about it until the next day. Weight loss tends to be slow and steady, a half to one-and-a-half pounds (0.2 to 0.7 kg) per week even though most dieters lose more in the first week. That's too slow to satisfy some folks.

That's a few of the reasons I devised the Ketogenic Mediterranean Diet.

VERY-LOW-CARBOHYDRATE DIETING

Another thumbnail sketch, this time for very-low-carbohydrate dieting. There are many different plans but they tend to share certain characteristics. If you're familiar with the Induction Phase of *Dr. Atkins New Diet Revolution*, you already know what I'm talking about.

Very-low-carb diets restrict carbohydrate consumption to 50 or fewer grams a day. This totally eliminates or drastically reduces some of our favorite foods, such as grains, beans, starchy vegetables (corn, potatoes, peas, etc), milk, and sugar. Nor can you have products made from these, such as bread, cookies, pies, cakes, potato and corn chips, and candy. You eat meat, eggs, fish, chicken, cheese, nuts, low-carb vegetables (e.g., salad greens, broccoli, green beans, cauliflower), and oils. Total calorie consumption is not restricted; you count carb grams rather than calories.

This is a radical change in eating for most people.

Numerous recent studies have demonstrated superior weight-loss results with very-low-carb diets as compared to traditional calorie-restricted diets. Weight loss is often faster and more consistently in the range of one or two pounds (0.5 to 0.9 kg) a week. Very-low-carb dieters have less trouble with hunger. If you do get hungry, there's always something you can eat. From a practical, day-to-day viewpoint, these diets can be easier to follow, with a bit less regimentation than calorie-restricted plans.

Sounds great! So why aren't very-low-carb diets used more often? Many dieters can't live with the restrictions. Your body may rebel against the switch from a carbohydrate-based energy metabolism to one based on fats. Most of us live in a society or sub-culture in which carbohydrates are everywhere and they're cheap; temptation is never-ending.

Just as calorie-restricted diets aren't for everybody, neither are very-low-carb diets. Some people respond to one or the other of the diet styles, others do well with either. With dieting, a one-size-fits-all approach is not the best. If it's safe, why not give folks a choice?

I've been an advocate of the traditional Mediterranean diet for the general public for over a decade. By "diet" in this context, I mean a person's usual way of eating, not a weight-loss program. In 2009, I took a close look at the individual components of the traditional Mediterranean diet and noted that many of them could be incorporated into a very-low-carbohydrate weight-loss diet. My idea was to combine the health benefits of the Mediterranean diet with the potential weight-loss benefits of very-low-carb diets. The result is the Ketogenic Mediterranean Diet.

ADVANCED OR KETOGENIC MEDITERRANEAN: HOW DO I CHOOSE?

Perhaps you have a strong preference already, just based on the thumbnail sketches. Don't ignore your intuition, but consider some other factors. Remember, you're not making an irrevocable lifelong decision. If your first choice doesn't suit you, try the other. Both plans work if you follow them. Some of my patients flip back and forth from one to the other, depending on their goals.

CHOOSE THE ADVANCED MEDITERRANEAN DIET IF . . .

- you want to capture the proven maximal health benefits of the Mediterranean diet
- you're a conservative, traditional type of person
- slower weight loss is acceptable
- you have any doubts about your underlying healthiness and strength
- you still believe that dietary total fat, saturated fat, and cholesterol promote heart and vascular disease
- you have gout, chronic kidney disease, or major chronic liver disease
- you just know you can't restrict carbohydrates drastically

- you've already tried and failed very-low-carb diets
- you don't like fish
- you enjoy the ultimate in variety

CHOOSE THE KETOGENIC MEDITERRANEN DIET IF . . .

- the potential for faster and easier weight loss appeals to you
- you're certain you're completely healthy and vigorous
- you think you can live with major carbohydrate restriction
- you've done well with very-low-carb eating in the past
- you prefer less regimentation
- you've suffered much hunger on calorie-restricted diets in the past
- you're not going to exercise
- you love salads and vinaigrettes
- you enjoy a glass of wine
- you don't have gout, chronic kidney disease, or major chronic liver disease

My gut feeling is that eating closer to the traditional Mediterranean diet, as opposed to very-low-carb eating, is probably the healthier way to go long-term. But we don't really know for sure. The two styles have never been compared head-to-head in a well-designed, multi-year, scientific study to answer the question: which is healthier? Unfortunately, we'll probably never see such a study done in our lifetimes.

6

The Ketogenic Mediterranean Diet

INTRODUCTION

I originally devised the very-low-carbohydrate Ketogenic Mediterranean Diet specifically for my patients
with one or more of the following conditions:
- type 2 diabetes
- prediabetes
- metabolic syndrome

As it turns out, the Ketogenic Mediterranean Diet
also works quite well for otherwise healthy people
who are just overweight or obese.

"Metabolic syndrome" may be a new term for you.
It's a constellation of clinical factors that are associated with increased future risk of type 2 diabetes
and atherosclerotic complications such as heart attack and stroke. One in six Americans has metabol-

ic syndrome. Diagnosis requires at least three of the following five conditions:

1. high blood pressure (130/85 or higher, or using a high blood pressure medication)
2. low HDL cholesterol: under 40 mg/dl (1.03 mmol/l) in a man, under 50 mg/dl (1.28 mmol/l) in a women (or either sex taking a cholesterol-lowering drug)
3. triglycerides over 150 mg/dl (1.70 mmol/l) (or taking a cholesterol-lowering drug)
4. abdominal fat: waist circumference 40 inches (102 cm) or greater in a man, 35 inches (89 cm) or greater in a woman
5. fasting blood glucose over 100 mg/dl (5.55 mmol/l)

Metabolic syndrome and simple excess weight often share a common trait: *impaired carbohydrate metabolism.* Overtime, excessive carbohydrate consumption can turn overweight and metabolic syndrome into prediabetes, then type 2 diabetes.

Diabetes and prediabetes always involve impaired carbohydrate metabolism: ingested carbs are not handled by the body in a healthy fashion, leading to high blood sugars and, eventually, poisonous complications.

In their 2011 book, *The Art and Science of Low Carbohydrate Living,* Drs. Jeff Volek and Stephen Phinney blame our epidemic of overweight on "carbohydrate intolerance." That's a more succinct way of saying "impaired carbohydrate metabolism."

You may recall from an earlier chapter Gary Taubes' explanation as to why we get fat: excessive carbohydrate consumption, leading to high insulin release by the pancrease, leading to build-up of fat tissue.

In other words, the carbohydrate/insulin theory of obesity.

The key feature of the Ketogenic Mediterranean Diet is carbohydrate restriction, which directly addresses impaired carbohydrate metabolism naturally.

My primary goal with this program—the world's first very-low-carb Mediterranean diet—is to reap the health benefits of Mediterranean-style eating while losing excess fat weight.

Secondary goals, which may not apply to you, are cure of metabolic syndrome and control of blood sugars in diabetics and prediabetics. Diabetics taking medications to control blood sugars may need to reduce drug dosages drastically. This should only be done under the supervision of a personal physician familiar with all medical details of the person with diabetes. You can find details about use of the Ketogenic Mediterranean Diet in diabetics in my book, *Conquer Diabetes and Prediabetes: The Low-Carb Mediterranean Diet* or at
http://DiabeticMediterraneanDiet.com.

WHY "KETOGENIC"?

Your body gets nearly all its energy either from fats, or from carbohydrates like glucose and glycogen. In people eating normally, 60% of their energy at rest comes from fats. In a ketogenic diet, the carbohydrate content of the diet is so low that the body has to break down even more of its fat to supply energy needed by most tissues. Fat breakdown generates ketone bodies in the bloodstream. Hence, "ketogenic diet." Also called "very-low-carb diets," ketogenic diets have been around for over a hundred years.

Ketogenic diets have several practical advantages over other diets (disputed by some authorities):

- simplicity
- almost unlimited access to many high-protein and fatty foods
- less trouble with hunger
- better short-term weight loss than many other diets (long-term, too?)
- lower blood sugar levels, which is important to people with diabetes, prediabetes, and metabolic syndrome
- reduced insulin levels in people who often have elevated levels (hyperinsulinemia), which may help reduce chronic diseases like type 2 diabetes, high blood pressure, some cancers, and coronary heart disease
- higher levels of HDL cholesterol and lower triglycerides, which may reduce risk of heart disease
- it obviously works well for a significant portion of the overweight population, but not for everybody
- better adherence to the program compared with other diets, at least for the short-term

WHY "MEDITERRANEAN"?

For years, the Mediterranean diet has been widely recognized as the healthiest diet for the general population. See the Introduction for details. The enduring popularity of the Mediterranean diet is attributable to three things:

1. Taste
2. Variety
3. Health benefits

(In this context, I'm using "diet" to refer to the usual food and drink of a person, not a weight-loss program.)

The traditional Mediterranean diet is rich in olive oil, fresh fruits and vegetables, nuts, fish, wine, whole grains, cheese, and yogurt, with minimal red meat. It's heavily influenced by the cuisines of Greece and southern Italy. See the Introduction for details about Mediterranean diet composition.

The scientist most responsible for the popularity of the diet, Ancel Keys, thought the heart-healthy aspects of the diet were related to low saturated fat consumption. He also thought the lower blood cholesterol levels in Mediterranean populations (at least Italy and Greece) had something to do with it, too. Dietary saturated fat does tend to raise cholesterol levels.

Even if Keys was wrong (and I think he was) about saturated fat and cholesterol levels being positively associated with heart disease, numerous studies indicate that the Mediterranean diet is one of the healthiest around. The research involved eight countries on three continents, so it's not just a Mediterranean climate or geography effect.

WHAT'S WRONG WITH PURE MEDITERRANEAN?

The traditional Mediterranean diet derives most of its calories from carbohydrates: anywhere from 45 to 60% of total energy. If the carbohydrate/insulin theory of obesity is correct, all those carbs could lead to excessive insulin release, leading in turn to storage of calories as fat tissue. For those trying to lose weight, the insulin could impair the ability to turn that fat into weightless energy.

The Ketogenic Mediterranean Diet removes most of the carbohydrates in the traditional Mediterranean diet, lowering insulin levels, allowing fat tissue to break down and supply us with energy. The very-low-carb Ketogenic Mediterranean Diet is also consistent with Volek and Phinney's "carbohydrate intolerance" model of overweight.

Despite an emphasis on carb-rich bread, pasta, fruits, legumes, and certain vegetables, the traditional Mediterranean diet has several healthy components compatible with a very-low-carb eating style:

- olive oil
- nuts and seeds
- low-carbohydrate vegetables
- low-carbohydrate fruits
- eggs
- chicken
- meat
- wine
- fish
- cheese
- Mediterranean spices

WHAT ABOUT WINE?

For centuries, the healthier populations in the Mediterranean region have enjoyed wine in light to moderate amounts, usually with meals. Epidemiologic studies there and in other parts of the world have associated reasonable alcohol consumption with prolonged life span, reduced coronary artery disease, diminished Alzheimer and other dementias, and possibly fewer strokes.

What's a "reasonable" amount of alcohol? An old medical school joke is that a "heavy drinker" is anyone who drinks more than the doctor does. Light to moderate alcohol consumption is generally considered to be one or fewer drinks per day for a woman, two or fewer drinks per day for a man. One drink is 5 ounces (150 ml) of wine, 12 ounces (355 ml) of beer, or 1.5 ounces (45 ml) of 80 proof distilled spirits (e.g., vodka, whiskey, gin). The optimal health-promoting type of alcohol is unclear. I tend to favor wine, a time-honored component of the Mediterranean diet. Red wine in particular is a rich source of resveratrol, which is thought to be a major contributor to the cardioprotective benefits associated with light to moderate alcohol consumption. Grape juice may be just as good; it's too soon to tell.

I have no intention of overselling the benefits of alcohol. If you are considering habitual alcohol as a food, be aware that the health benefits are still somewhat debatable. Consumption of three or more alcoholic drinks per day is clearly associated with a higher risk of breast cancer in women. Even one or two drinks daily may slightly increase the risk. Folic acid supplementation might mitigate the risk. If you are a woman and breast cancer runs in your family, strongly consider abstinence. Be cautious if there are alcoholics in your family; you may have inherited the predisposition. If you take any medications or have chronic medical conditions, check with your personal physician first. For those drinking above light to moderate levels, alcohol is clearly perilous. Higher dosages can cause hypertension, liver disease, heart failure, certain cancers, and other medical problems. And psychosocial problems. And legal problems. And death. Heavy drinkers have higher rates of violent and accidental death. Alcoholism is often fatal.

You should not drink alcohol if you:
- have a history of alcohol abuse or alcoholism
- have liver or pancreas disease
- are pregnant or trying to become pregnant
- may have the need to operate dangerous equipment or machinery, such as an automobile, while under the influence of alcohol
- have a demonstrated inability to limit yourself to acceptable intake levels
- have personal prohibitions due to religious, ethical, or other reasons.

POTENTIAL PROBLEMS WITH VERY-LOW-CARB EATING

Long-term effects of a very-low-carb or ketogenic diet in most people are unclear. Overall health outcomes may be better or worse; we just don't know for sure yet. Perhaps some people gain a clear benefit, while others—with different metabolisms and genetic make-up—are worse off.

If the diet results in major weight loss that lasts, we may see longer life span, less type 2 diabetes, less cancer, less heart disease, less high blood pressure, and fewer of the other obesity-related medical conditions.

Ketogenic diets are generally higher in protein, total fat, saturated fat, and cholesterol than some other diets, at least in terms of percentages. Some authorities are concerned this may increase the risk of coronary heart disease and stroke; the latest evidence indicates otherwise (see Selected References at the back of the book).

Some authorities worry that ketogenic diets have the potential to cause kidney stones, osteoporosis (thin, brittle bones), gout, deficiency of vitamins and minerals, and may worsen existing kidney disease. Others disagree.

It's clear that compliance with very-low-carb diets is difficult to maintain for six to 12 months. In other words, it's hard to stick with it. Many folks can't do it for more than a couple weeks. Potential long-term effects, therefore, haven't come into play for most users. When used for weight loss, regain of lost weight is a problem, but regain is a major issue with all weight-loss programs. I anticipate that the majority of non-diabetics who try a ketogenic diet will stay on it for only one to six months. After that, more carbohydrates can be added to gain the potential long-term benefits of additional fruits and vegetables, legumes, and whole grains.

People with type 2 diabetes or prediabetes may be so pleased with the metabolic effects of the ketogenic diet that they'll stay on it long-term.

MORE ON CARBOHYDRATE INTOLERANCE

Most overweight and obese folks must remember that their bodies do not, and cannot, handle dietary carbs in a normal, healthy fashion. This applies especially to the fattening carbs: sugars and refined starches. In a way, carbs are toxic to the overweight and obese, leading to increased risk of weight-related medical problems.

Most overweight people simply don't tolerate carbs in the diet like other people. If you don't tolerate something, you have to give it up, or at least cut way back on it. Lactose-intolerant individuals give up milk and other lactose sources. Celiac disease patients don't tolerate gluten, so they give up wheat and other sources of gluten. One of every five high blood pressure patients can't handle normal levels of salt in the diet; they have to cut back or their pressure's too high. Patients with phenylketonuria don't tolerate phenylalanine and have to restrict foods that contain it. If you're allergic to penicillin, you have to give it up. If you don't tolerate carbs, you have to give them up or cut way back. I'm sorry.

PRECAUTIONS AND DISCLAIMER

The ideas and suggestions in this book are provided as general educational information only and should not be construed as medical advice or care. Information herein is meant to complement, not replace, any advice or information from your personal health professional. All matters regarding your health require supervision by a personal physician or other appropriate health professional familiar with your current health status. Always consult your personal physician before making any dietary or exercise changes. Steve Parker, M.D., and the publisher disclaim any liability or warranties of any kind arising directly or indirectly from use of this diet. If any medical problems develop, always consult your personal physician. Only your physician can provide you medical advice. You should not follow this diet if you are a child, pregnant or lactating, have alcoholism or history of alcohol abuse, have abnormal liver or kidney function, or have gout or a high uric acid blood level. Your physician may have to adjust medication dosages—particularly blood pressure pills and diabetic drugs—if you follow this diet.

LET'S GET STARTED!

The Ketogenic Mediterranean Diet is a very-low-carb diet providing 20 to 40 grams of digestible carbohydrate daily. It's designed for loss of excess body fat and control of high blood sugars. "Digestible carbo-hydrate" is the total carbohydrate grams minus the fiber grams of carbohydrate that you can't digest and utilize as an energy source.

For you nutrition science geeks, here's the macro-nutrient breakdown. Of the total calories eaten, 7–10% are from carbohydrate, 55–65% are from fat, 22–30% are from protein, and 5–10% are from alcohol.

You'll find a three-page printable version of the basic Ketogenic Mediterranean Diet (KMD) here: http://advancedmediterraneandiet.com/printabledocuments.html

HERE'S WHAT YOU'LL EAT:

1) Unlimited fish, meat, chicken, turkey, eggs, shrimp, lobster
2) Fish, at least 4 oz (115 g) daily
3) Olive oil, virgin or extra-virgin, at least 2–3 tbsp (30–45 ml) daily
4) Nuts and seeds, 1 oz (28 g) daily
5) Vegetables, up to 14 oz (400 g) daily
6) Wine, 6–12 fl oz (180–360 ml) daily (see alternatives in Miscellaneous Comments)
7) Cheese, up to 3 oz (85 g) daily, optional
8) Daily supplements:
   • 1 or 2 plain Centrum multivita-min/multimineral supplements (two if over 250 lb or 114 kg)
   • Magnesium oxide 250 mg
   • Calcium carbonate 500 mg elemental calcium (500 mg twice daily if over 250 lb or 114 kg)
   • Extra vitamin D to reach total of 1,000–1,200 IU (each Centrum has 400 IU)
   • Potassium gluconate 2,750 mg (450 mg

elemental potassium) or Morton Salt
Substitute (potassium chloride) ¼ tsp (1.2 g)
- If prone to constipation: sugar-free Metamucil powder 1–2 rounded tsp (5.8–11.6 g) in water
- At least three quarts or liters of water

What makes it Mediterranean? Natural whole foods, fish, olive oil, nuts, wine, cheese, spices.

What's not Mediterranean? Unlimited meat and animal proteins, and absence of most sweet fruits, high-carbohydrate vegetables, potatoes, grains, legumes, pasta, honey, and yogurt. These may come later.

You can track your consumption of the major foods with the "KMD & LCMD Daily Log" available for free at http://advancedmediterraneandiet.com/printabledo cuments.html

See chapter seven for "A Week of Meals" consistent with the Ketogenic Mediterranean Diet. Or just use your imagination while following the guidelines above.

WARNING

Wine and other alcoholic beverages are dangerous. You should not drink wine or any alcohol if you have a history of alcohol abuse or alcoholism, have liver or pancreas disease, are pregnant or trying to become pregnant, may have the need to operate dangerous equipment or machinery—such as driving a car—while under the influence of alcohol, or have demonstrated inability to limit yourself to acceptable intake levels.

FOOD CATEGORY COMMENTS:

1. Protein Group

This includes fish, meat, chicken, turkey, eggs, shrimp, lobster, and fried pork skins. Try to avoid overly processed protein products; aim for pure and simple. Processed meats may have added carbohydrates, nitrites, and other chemicals you don't need. Canned products are OK. *Eat until full or satisfied, not stuffed.*

2. Fish

Canned fish may be more affordable and convenient. Cold-water fatty fish have more of the healthy omega-3 fatty acids: trout, salmon, sardines, mackerel, albacore/white tuna, herring, swordfish, halibut, sea bass. If you're pregnant, trying to become pregnant, or a nursing mother, avoid eating king mackerel, swordfish, shark, and tilefish (sold as golden snapper or golden bass); these fish may contain amounts of mercury harmful to breast-fed infants and babies in the womb. If you eat lots of locally caught freshwater fish, especially if you are a women of childbearing age, check with your regional governmental authorities regarding contaminants. In the U.S., the appropriate state agency is usually the Health Department or Game and Fish Department. Note that adult medical problems attributable to chemical fish contamination are exceedingly rare in the U.S.

3. Olive oil

Use virgin or extra virgin oil in vinaigrette or other olive oil-based salad dressing. Sauté with it. Fry eggs and steak with it. Drink it straight if you want!

113

KMD

4. Nuts and Seeds

Almonds, walnuts, pecans, Brazil nuts, hazelnuts (filberts), macadamia nuts, peanuts (a legume), Spanish peanuts, pistachios, pine nuts, sunflower seeds, pumpkin seeds in shells. These average 3 g of digestible carbohydrate per ounce (28 g). Sunflower seeds, peanuts, and pistachios are the highest in carbs: 3.5 to 4 g per ounce (28 g). Sorry, no cashews.

5. Vegetables & Fruit

(A) Raw salad vegetables: lettuce, mushrooms, radishes, spinach, alfalfa sprouts, cucumber, tomato, scallions, parsley, jicama, arugula, endive, radicchio, chard, sweet peppers, avocado, olives (pickled green or ripe black), pickles (dill or sour, not sweet or "bread and butter"). Average digestible carbohydrate per 7 oz serving (200 g) is 5 g. The highest digestible carb counts are in scallions and jicama (8 g), and sweet peppers (7g).

(B) Solid vegetables, often cooked: snow peas, broccoli, summer squash, tomato, onion, cauliflower, eggplant, Brussels sprouts, asparagus, okra, sauerkraut (canned), green beans. These average 8 g of digestible carbohydrate per 7 oz serving (200 g). Onion is highest at 14 g. Weigh these before cooking.

6. Wine

Red wine (e.g., Burgundy, Cabernet Sauvignon, or Merlot) may be healthier than white (e.g., Sauvignon Blanc, Riesling, Pinot Grigio). One fl oz (30 ml) of wine has 1 g of carbohydrate.

114

7. Cheese

Real, regular cheese; not low-fat. Mozzarella, provolone, Swiss, cheddar, blue, Monterey, Colby, Brie, Parmesan, feta, Gouda, ricotta, cottage. These have 1 g carbohydrate per oz (28 g). Other cheeses have too many carbs.

MISCELLANEOUS COMMENTS:

Alternatives to wine (choose only one daily):
- Extra 200 g (7 oz) vegetables, and consider a grape extract supplement daily, or
- 20 g (0.7 oz) of dark chocolate (65-85% cacao) daily, or
- Beer, 12 fl oz (360 ml) daily, but must have under 10 g of carbs, or
- Distilled spirits (whiskey, rum, vodka, gin), 80 proof, 1.5 fl oz (45 ml) daily

Additional daily optional oils, spices, and condiments (unlimited unless noted):

Butter, plant oils (strongly favor olive oil), vinegar (cider, red wine, or distilled), balsamic vinegar (2 tsp or 10 ml daily), salt, pepper, genuine mayonnaise (not low-fat), yellow mustard (1 tbsp or 15 ml daily), salad dressing (with three or fewer grams of carbohydrate per 2 tbsp or 30 ml) (2 tbsp daily), Worcestershire sauce (1 tbsp or 15 ml), A.1. Steak Sauce (1 tbsp or 15 ml)

Prominent Mediterranean spices: paprika, cumin, turmeric, cinnamon, ginger (0.35 oz or 10 g raw root, or 2 tsp or 10 ml ground spice daily), coriander, anise, Spanish saffron, lemon or lime juice (2 tbsp or 30 ml daily), mint, parsley, garlic (3 cloves daily), dill pepper, and sumac

Tea and coffee in moderation are fine. Don't add milk to them; use full-fat cream or high-fat half-and-half.

All of the recommended supplements are readily available at supermarkets and pharmacies at a reasonable cost.

I recommend Centrum for people on the Ketogenic Mediterranean Diet. Why Centrum? It's been around for years and has a good reputation. It's widely available at a reasonable price. A different brand of multivitamin/multimineral supplement may be fine if it's close to Centrum's components. Since the composition of plain Centrum could change at any time (or be concocted differently in non-U.S. countries), listed below are the contents of the U.S. product in 2011. Here are the component amounts with "% Daily Values" in parentheses:

Vitamin A 3,5000 IU (70%), Vitamin C 60 mg (100%), Vitamin D 400 IU (100%), Vitamin E 30 IU (100%), Vitamin K 25 mcg (31%), Thiamin 1.5 mg (100%), Riboflavin 1.7 mg (100%), Niacin 20 mg (100%), Vitamin B6 2 mg (100%), Folic Acid 400 mcg (100%), Vitamin B12 6 mcg (100%), Biotin 30 mcg (10%), Pantothenic Acid 10 mg (100%), Calcium 200 mg (20%), Iron 18 mg (100%), Phosphorus 20 mg (2%), Iodine 150 mcg (100%), Magnesium 50 mg (13%), Zinc 11 mg (73%), Selenium 55 mcg (79%), Copper 0.5 mg (25%), Manganese 2.3 mg (115%), Chromium 35 mcg (29%), Molybdenum 45 mcg (60%), Chloride 72 mg (2%), Potassium 80 mg (2%), Boron 75 mcg, Nickel 5 mcg, Silicon 2 mg, Tin 10 mcg, Vanadium 10 mcg.

U.S. government authorities recommend Percent Daily Values for average non-pregnant healthy adults eating 2,000 calorie a day.

Need a sweet, crunchy treat? Metamucil Fiber Wafers (12 g each), two per week.

Don't just eat the same eight or 10 items—aim for great variety. For meal ideas, see chapter seven for a week of meals and special recipes.

You'll be eating lots of salad.

You'll need a scale to measure your vegetables and to follow the optional recipes in chapter seven.

To make your food shopping easier, you can print a grocery shopping list of all foods on the Ketogenic Mediterranean Diet when you visit this web page: http://advancedmediterraneandiet.com/printabledo cuments.html

WHAT COULD GO WRONG?

Very-low-carb ketogenic diets have been associated with headaches, bad breath, easy bruising, nausea, fatigue, aching, muscle cramps, constipation, and dizziness, among other symptoms. "Induction flu" may occur around days two through five, consisting of achiness, easy fatigue, and low energy. It usually clears up after a few days.

Very-low-carb ketogenic diets may have the potential to cause osteoporosis (thin, brittle bones), kidney stones, low blood pressure, constipation, gout, high uric acid in the blood, excessive loss of sodium and potassium in the urine, worsening of kidney disease, deficiency of calcium and vitamins A, B, C, and D, among other adverse effects.

Athletic individuals who perform vigorous exercise should expect a deterioration in performance levels during the first three to four weeks of any ketogenic very-low-carb diet. The body needs that time to adjust to burning mostly fat for fuel rather than carbohydrate.

Competitive weight-lifters or other anaerobic athletes (e.g., sprinters) may be hampered by the low muscle glycogen stores that accompany ketogenic diets. They may need more carbohydrates.

WHAT'S NEXT?

I recommend that anyone trying the Ketogenic Mediterranean Diet give it at least an eight to 12 week trial. Then evaluate whether it's time to move on to higher carbohydrate consumption. Remember, the KMD provides 20 to 40 grams of carbohydrate daily. Everyone has a different level of "carbohydrate intolerance" that leads to fat weight gain. It takes experimentation to find your personal intolerance level. Many people find that if they exceed 80 to 100 grams daily, they gain back the lost weight. See chapter 9 for advice on transitioning to higher carbohydrate consumption and long-term maintenance of weight loss.

7

Daily Life With Low-Carb Eating

I haven't scared you off yet, huh?

Great!

The very-low-carbohydrate program I've laid out presents some definite challenges, a few of which are unique. Think of them as opportunities for personal growth. But you don't have to go it alone, nor blaze any trails through uncharted territory. I'm here to help, as is a scattered online low-carb community.

This chapter will give you an approach to overcoming the common problems linked to low-carb eating. The coping mechanisms here are not exhaustive, and you'll need, at times, to figure out for yourself what works for you and your unique situation.

In order, here's what's ahead:

1. FIND MORE LOW-CARB RECIPES

Chapter seven has some low-carb recipes. Find many more at free low-carb websites and online forums, such as:
- The message boards at Low Carb Friends (http://www.lowcarbfriends.com)
- Active Low-Carbers Forum (http://forum.lowcarber.org)
- Laura Dolson's About.com: Low Carb Diets blog (http://lowcarbdiets.about.com)
- Chef Barrae has posted hundreds of low-carb recipes (including nutritional analysis) at her blog: Unrestricted Tastes on Restricted Diets: Distinctive Diabetic Recipes (http://chefbarrae.blogspot.com).
- Jennifer Eloff has authored numerous low-carb cookbooks, starting with her flagship, *Splendid Low-Carbing*, followed by four others in the same vein. Jennifer generously shares many of her fantastic recipes at her

blog, Splendid Low-Carbing. Most of her recipes include some nutrient analysis, such as carb and calorie counts. Jennifer has a particular interest in cooking with Splenda, helping you satisfy your sweet tooth. Find her blog at
(http://low-carb-news.blogspot.com/).

- DAR, a type 2 diabetic, offers her favorite low-carb recipes at http://dardreams.wordpress.com/. Nutrient analysis is limited to digestible carb grams, referred to as "net carbs."

- Dana Carpender has a number of great low-carb recipe books, such as the classic *500 Low-Carb Recipes*, as well as *200 Low-Carb Slow Cooker Recipes*, *15-Minute Low-Carb Recipes*, and *1001 Low-Carb Recipes*. Check out some of her free online recipes and purchase books at her blog, Hold the Toast! (http://holdthetoast.com/).

- All Day I Dream About Food (http://dreamaboutfood.blogspot.com/). Carolyn Ketchum, a blogger with prediabetes, shares her low-carb and/or gluten-free recipes.

Among the many low-carb cookbooks available, a great place to start is *Low-Carbing Among Friends*, Volume 1, by Jennifer Eloff, Maria Emmerich, Carolyn Ketchum, Lisa Marshall, and Kent Altena. All 325 recipes are both gluten-free and low-carb (10 or fewer grams per serving).

You need to know the digestible or *net carb grams* per serving of any recipe you try. If not provided for you, you can do a full nutritional analysis of any recipe at SELF-NutritionData
(http://nutritiondata.self.com/).

2. SHORT-TERM PHYSICAL EFFECTS

Very-low-carb eating is quite safe in the vast majority of generally healthy people. However, you need to be aware of minor problems that may crop up.

INDUCTION FLU

This refers to a sense of mild malaise, easy-fatigue, low energy, achiness, and dizziness that often affects people switching from a carbohydrate-based energy metabolism to fat-based. Some folks have the entire syndrome, others just parts. It starts on the second or third day of the diet and may last for several days, a week at the most. People with diabetes need to make sure the symptoms are not caused by low blood sugar by using their home glucose monitor.

Regarding low energy and easy fatigue, people who are used to exercising or working vigorously may notice that they can't perform at their prior workload, an effect that may be noticeable for two to four weeks. They may need to cut back the intensity of their work-outs temporarily. The first few weeks of very-low-carb eating are not a good time to start a vigorous exercise program.

Induction flu is temporary. It's proof that your body is going through a watershed moment. Try to tough it out. You'll be glad you did.

LEG CRAMPS

These occur commonly in the first few weeks or months. They tend to happen at night, even waking people from sleep. While not serious, they can be painful. Cramps are often prevented by taking additional supplemental magnesium, potassium, calcium, or a combination. If they persist, see your doctor for a blood test of these minerals.

A stretching exercise may prevent leg cramps: 1) Stand about two or three feet away from a wall (measured at the toes) and keep your feet planted in one spot, 2) lean forward against the wall and use your outstretched arms and hands to keep your body from hitting the wall, 3) keeping your trunk and legs in a straight line, bend your elbows to let your head approach the wall, 4) notice the slight tensing and stretching of the calf muscles (this may be slightly uncomfortable but shouldn't be painful), 5) hold that position for 10 seconds, 6) then stand up straight and relax a while, 7) repeat steps 1 through 5 for five or ten times. For nocturnal leg cramps, do this stretching just before bedtime.

CONSTIPATION OR DIARRHEA

If a bowel problem occurs, it's more likely to be constipation related to lower-than-usual fiber consumption. Others have the opposite problem, diarrhea. Go figure. You might be able to identify a specific food causing symptoms, such as cheese and constipation. Eliminate or cut back on the offending item. Sugar-free Metamucil powder (one teaspoon in water) once or twice daily usually resolves constipation. Or you could concentrate on the higher fiber vegetables.

LOW BLOOD SUGAR

Since ingested carbohydrates are normally the main source of blood sugar, cutting back drastically tends to reduce blood sugar levels, even in people who don't have diabetes or prediabetes. Symptoms of low blood sugar (hypoglycemia) are rare in healthy people starting a ketogenic diet. But hypoglycemia is much more common and potentially serious in diabetics taking certain medications.

LOW BLOOD PRESSURE

The Ketogenic Mediterranean Diet is relatively low in salt, which may explain why low blood pressure can occur. If you take drugs to lower your blood pressure, the dosage my need to be reduced to prevent excessively low blood pressure. Symptoms of low blood pressure include dizziness, lightheadedness, weakness, fainting, and fatigue. Note the similarity to induction flu. You may notice these only when going from sitting to standing, or from lying to standing.

If low blood pressure is causing the symptom, we usually find a systolic blood pressure under 90 mmHg. "Systolic pressure" is the top or first number in a blood pressure reading such as 125/85 (systolic pressure is 125). The only way to tell if the aforementioned symptoms are related to blood pressure is to check a blood pressure with an accurate monitor, which most of us don't have at home or work. Perhaps you could borrow a friend's. Alternatively, check your blood pressure at your doctor's office or one of the free machines in many pharmacies and supermarkets. In those settings, a systolic pressure under 100 mmHg, even if you feel fine, suggests that your pressure at other times is under 90. Low blood pressures often responds to an increase in salt and water consumption, such as half a teaspoon daily mixed in water or used on food.

3. SHOPPING

Finding food for the Ketogenic Mediterranean Diet shouldn't be a problem. Specific recommended foods are readily available at supermarkets. People committed long-term to the low-carb way of eating often get into baking or cooking with low-carb components that may be a bit harder to find. An example is almond flour, used as a substitute for wheat flour in baking cookies and pastries, among other things. You may find low-carb products at local stores or available on the Internet (e.g., Netrition.com).

You'll find a grocery shopping list for the Ketogenic and Low-Carb Mediterranean Diets (more on LCMD later) at this URL:
http://advancedmediterraneandiet.com/printabledo
cuments.html

How to choose a fresh fish for cooking:

1. Sniff it. Pass if it smells fishy, nasty, or pungent.
2. Check for clear, dark eyes. Pass if eyes are dull gray and sunken.
3. Does it look or feel slimy? Take a pass.
4. Skin should be moist and shiny, almost metallic.
5. Flesh should be firm, not mushy. Press it with your finger—it shouldn't leave an imprint.
6. Look for bright red gills.
7. Cook within a day or two.

Keep your refrigerator and cupboards stocked with the foods you'll be eating, particularly if others in your household are eating regular high-carb foods that will tempt you.

4. DINING OUT

You'll be tempted to return to "normal" high-carb eating especially when you're away from your home's well-stocked cupboards and refrigerator. Be ready to deal with it.

One option is to take your food with you. For road trips, take nuts, dark chocolate, canned fish and meat, vegetables, an ice cooler stocked with cheese, condiments, vegetables, and your favorite low-carb or no-carb drinks. (My family likes to stay at motels with "free breakfast," but that too often means the only low-carb offerings are butter and half-n-half coffee creamer.)

Buffets will have several low-carb options for you.

Fast-food restaurants also offer several low-carb options. Order a burger and throw away the bun. Or they may build the burger for you wrapped in lettuce instead of bread. Eat the topping of pizza, not the bread. Fancy salads topped with chicken or beef are commonly available. Nearly all fast-food restaurants provide nutritional analysis for menu items; ask for it if you aren't sure of the carb count.

5. CHEATING

Let's face it: everybody cheats on diets.

It's easier to deal with the truth when you recognize the truth. It's not going to be the end of the world if you go "off plan" for one or two days a year and just eat like everyone else around you. I'm not suggesting pigging out as if you were at a decadent ancient Roman feast. Just eat reasonable amounts of regular, carb-rich foods. You'll probably gain a pound or two (up to a kilogram). Returning to a strict Keto-genic Mediterranean Diet and exercising a little more for a few days will usually resolve the extra weight.

A more common issue is that someone has a crav-ing for a particular food and can't live with the pos-sibility of never eating it again. For instance, I love apple pie and Cinnabon cinnamon rolls; I'd get de-pressed if I could never again have them. So what I'll do, perhaps every couple months, is have the cinnamon roll (730 calories and 115 grams of carb!) or a large serving of apple pie *instead of a meal*. Call it a "cheat meal." I eat low-carb, maybe even lower than usual, for the remainder of that day. What about eating your usual three daily meals *plus* the cinnamon roll, and just burn off the extra calories with exercise? Sounds logical. But a 150-pound person (68 kg) would need to jump rope for four and a half hours to burn 730 calories. I won't do that, and you won't either.

Cheat days and cheat meals don't work for every-one. Think about alcoholics who have stopped drinking. Standard advice from addiction specialists is that alcoholics should *never* again drink alcohol. I agree. Not even a sip. Probably not even non-alcoholic "beer." That's because it's too tempting and could trigger a drinking binge that could be life-threatening. A few people are that way with carbo-hydrates. You could say they're addicted, or carbo-holics. They shouldn't have cheat days or cheat meals. Does this apply to you? Only you can answer that.

6. SWEET CRAVINGS

If sweets are your downfall, be aware that cravings tend to dissipate after several months of low-carbing. It may take up to a year. Unfortunately, that doesn't happen for everyone.

If your cravings persist and you can't resist them, your best option is non-caloric artificial sweeteners, sometimes known as sugar substitutes. Examples are sucralose, aspartame, sorbitol, erythritol, and stevia. Several of these can be used in cooking and baking.

Online low-carb recipe repositories will have many sweet options. Or use off-the-shelf prepared items from grocery stores. Try sugar-free gelatin or sugar-free hard candy.

I have no objection if you wish to drink one or two diet soda pops a day. Water may be better for you.

7. HOLIDAYS

Holidays like Thanksgiving (in the U.S.) and Christmas present major temptations to folks trying to limit carb consumption. It's easier to stay "on plan" if you don't socialize much, but most of us visit relatives or others, and the temptation to eat like everyone else is great and often irresistible.

Sometimes people almost "force" carbs on you. Diabetics and prediabetics can say, "No, thanks. My doctor has me on a special diet," and that should be the end of it. Others can say, "I'm fine, thank you. I just feel better if I eat a different way," or, "I'm fine, thank you. I'm not hungry right now." Best of all, say "No, thanks. I'm on Dr. Parker's Ketogenic Mediterranean Diet. It's great; let me tell you about it!"

Another option is to cheat on the diet.

8. HUNGER

If you get hungry between meals, choose an item from the "unlimited" foods list and see if that helps. Or eat cheese, up to three ounces a day. A can of tuna or a couple hard-boiled eggs may not be your traditional snacks, but they aren't likely to blow your weight management plan compared to a bag of corn chips or handful of cookies.

9. RECORD-KEEPING

Record-keeping is critical, at least early on. Keep a daily log. Design your own or use my online form (see below). Note 1) your consumption of the major food items, 2) any transgressions, 3) anything that may have precipitated transgressions, 4) a description of exercise done, 5) daily weight, 6) anything else you deem pertinent. Note changes in blood lipids if they're an issue. The "KMD & LCMD Daily Log" is available free at
http://advancedmediterraneandiet.com/printabledo cuments.html.

If desired, you can pretty easily keep track of your daily consumption online at SELF-NutritionData. The web address is http://nutritiondata.self.com/. First, register your free membership. Then go to the "My ND" section near the top of the page and click on "My Recipes." Make each of your days a single recipe with a title such as "LCMD Day 1." Enter everything you eat in the course of a day. Remember to click "Save" before you leave that day's recipe. At the end of the day, choose the "Save and Analyze" button. You'll get a comprehensive nutritional analysis of that day's consumption.

And I mean *comprehensive*: overall percentages of carbohydrate, protein, and fat, along with total calories and 40 or 50 vitamins, minerals, and other nutrients.

If you're going to do this for more than a couple days, use the "My Foods" feature and you'll end up saving time. An exercise like this (essentially a food diary) over four or five days is also helpful in figuring out why weight loss may have stalled or blood sugars are getting higher. Carb consumption often creeps up unnoticed, and at a certain point will sabotage the best-laid plans.

You can do similar record-keeping and nutritional analysis at FitDay (http://fitday.com/). FitDay also helps you easily track your weight and exercise and estimate calories burned exercising. It's definitely worth a look. It's free.

Yet another good free option for record-keeping is Calorie Count (http://caloriecount.about.com/).

Both Calorie Count and FitDay have active community forums for weight-loss support and education.

10. WEIGHT-LOSS TIPS

Plan on grocery shopping, meal preparation, and taking meals to your workplace.

Record-keeping is often the key to success. For options, see the section immediately preceding this.

Accountability is another key to success. Consider documenting your program and progress on a free website such as FitDay, SparkPeople, 3FatChicks, or others. If your initiation to low-carb eating is a major undertaking (and it should be) consider blogging about your adventure on a free platform such as Wordpress or Blogger. Such a public commitment may be just what you need to keep you motivated.

Do you have a friend or spouse who wants to lose weight? Start the same program at the same time and support each other. That's built-in accountability.

If you tend to over-eat, floss and brush your teeth after you're full. You'll be less likely to go back for more anytime soon.

Eat at least two or three meals daily. Eat breakfast routinely. Skipping meals may lead to uncontrollable overeating later on. On the other hand, ignore the diet gurus who say you *must* eat every two or three hours.

For at least a few times, try presenting your food on attractive dishes with a decorative place mat. Eat slowly to allow yourself time to enjoy your food and to appreciate when you're full.

Eat meals at a leisurely pace, chewing and enjoying each bite thoroughly before swallowing. Traditional Mediterranean meals are a time for socializing, too. Don't eat while watching TV.

Plan to give yourself a specific reward for every 10 pounds (4.5 kg) of weight lost. You know what you like. Consider a weekend get-away, a trip to the beauty salon, jewelry, an evening at the theater, a professional massage, home entertainment equipment, new clothes, etc.

Carefully consider when would be a good time to start your new lifestyle. It should be a period of low or usual stress. Bad times would be Thanksgiving Day, Christmas/New Years' holiday, the first day of a Caribbean cruise, and during a divorce.

If you know you've eaten enough at a meal to satisfy your nutritional requirements yet you still feel hungry, drink a large glass of water and wait a while. Or try a sugar-free psyllium fiber supplement such as Metamucil (3 grams of fiber per rounded teaspoon or 5 ml) with 8 ounces (240 ml) of water.

Limit television to less than two hours a day.

If a food item isn't on the list of food choices, don't keep it in the house unless you're sure it won't tempt you beyond your limits.

Maintain a consistent eating pattern throughout the week and year.

Control emotional eating.

Weigh frequently: daily during active weight-loss efforts and during the first two months of your maintenance-of-weight-loss phase. After that, cut back to weekly weights if you want. Daily weights will remind you how hard you worked to achieve your goal.

Be aware that you might regain five or 10 pounds (2.3 or 4.5 kg) of fat now and then. You probably will. Don't freak out. It's human nature. You're not a failure; you're human. But draw the line and get back on the old Ketogenic Mediterranean Diet for one or two months. Analyze and learn from the episode. Why did it happen? Slipping back into your old ways? Slacking off on exercise? Too many special occasion feasts or cheat days? Allowing junk food or non-essential carbs back into the house?

Learn which food item is your nemesis, the food that consistently torpedoes your resolve to eat right. For example, mine is anything sweet. Remember an old ad campaign for a potato chip: "Betcha can't eat just one!"? Well, I can't eat just one cookie. So I don't get started. I might eat one if it's the last one available. Or I satisfy my sweet craving with a diet soda, piece of dark chocolate, or sugar-free gelatin. Just as a recovering alcoholic can't drink any alcohol, perhaps you should totally abstain from...? You know your own personal gastronomic Achilles heel. Or heels. Experiment with various strategies for vanquishing your nemesis.

Tell your housemates you're on a special diet and ask for their support. You may also need to tell your co-workers and others with whom you spend significant time. If they care about you, they'll be careful not to tempt you off the diet.

Gnawing hunger is infrequent with the Ketogenic Mediterranean program. It may be a sign that you're exercising excessively. Try cutting back on physical activity, and accept a slower rate of weight loss.

Use a food scale and measuring devices to improve your compliance with portion sizes, especially during the first month. Thereafter you may be able to judge portion size by eye and feel.

One ounce (28 g) of cheese is about the size of a domino.

An ounce (28 g) of nuts is about a quarter of a cup, or a heap of nuts in the palm of your hand, not covering your fingers.

Fish and poultry may be a little more healthful for you than red meat.

Regular meat products may be a little healthier than processed meats like bacon, bologna and other luncheon meats, pre-cooked commercial sausages, etc.

As long as a food is low-carb, don't go for the low-fat version. For instance, low-fat yogurt is over-loaded with carbohydrates compared to the full-fat version.

Do your grocery shopping from a list.

For help with basic culinary skills, peruse these books: How *to Cook Everything: Simple Recipes for Great Food*, by Mark Bittman; *Joy of Cooking: 75th Anniversary Edition*, by Irma S. Rombauer, Marion Rombauer Becker, and Ethan Becker; *Betty Crocker Cookbook: Everything You Need to Know to Cook Today*.

11. SOCIAL ISSUES

AGAINST THE GRAIN OF A CARB-CENTRIC CULTURE

There was a time in my life that I just loved whole grain bread, pizza, and pasta. I couldn't imagine life without them. As an experiment, I went an entire year eating low-carb, without whole grain bread, pizza, and pasta. After that, I didn't miss them much at all. I realized I could easily have a happy, healthy, fulfilling, life without whole grain bread, pizza, and pasta. If you told me I had a medical condition that would worsen if I ate them, I could easily live without them and not complain.

During that same experimental year, I cut way back on my consumption of sweet fruits, starchy vegetables, and sweets (cookies, cakes, candy bars, pies). After the year was up, I didn't miss the sweet fruits and starchy vegetables, although I did miss my sweet things. I could see living the rest of my life without sweet fruits and starchy vegetables. Giving up apple pie and Cinnabon cinnamon rolls would be tougher.

That's just my experience, but I'm not alone. I wouldn't ask you to give up many of your beloved carbohydrates if I didn't know it was possible, and that others had done it successfully. The trade-offs for many of us will be improved health and slimmer waistlines.

The odd thing about the Ketogenic Mediterranean Diets is that it goes against the grain (pun intended) of the Western food culture that prominently features carbohydrates. Anyone following the diet is immediately in a strange position, surrounded continuously with opportunities and inducements to consume carbs. Especially nutrient-depleted, highly refined carbs such as white bread, sugar, flour, fruit juice, potato and corn chips (crisps), high fructose corn syrup, and soda pop.

It's difficult to swim against the tide in such a carb-cenric culture, especially when you've been enjoying carbs for 30 or 40 years before they finally caused your overweight problem. Old habits are hard to break. Food preferences are deeply ingrained from an early age.

One way to counteract that cultural pull is to take to heart the medical consequences of progressive overweight and obesity as outlined in chapter two. How do you motivate someone today to make a radical change in behavior that may not have a health-related pay-off for another decade or more? Education is the only tactic I know that works consistently. People are more receptive when they're hospitalized with diabetic symptoms and blood sugars are elevated to four times normal. Even then change is often a struggle.

Low-carb eating increasingly will be seen as viable and healthful as news of recent scientific developments becomes mainstream. Low-carbing will be easier to maintain then, as more folks get on board.

ONLINE SUPPORT

If you feel lonely and odd eating very-low-carb, you'll find copious online support at the Low Carb Friends message boards (http://lowcarbfriends.com/) and Active Low-Carbers Forum (http://forum.lowcarber.org/). There are plenty of low-carbers also on the forums at FitDay, Spark-People, and 3FatChicks.

PARTIES AND HOLIDAY MEALS

In general, I think it's a good idea to let those around you know that you're eating low-carb. I understand there may be good reasons to keep it a secret, however. If you're not in charge of the food, let the host know you'll be focusing on meat, chicken, eggs, fish, cheese, and low-carb vegetables. The meats are usually main courses anyway. You'll simply not be eating many of the side dishes like bread, potatoes, corn, peas, and desserts. If you're the host, you'll probably want to provide your guests, especially children, with the usual high-carb fare. With some experience, you could serve adults a delicious low-carb feast without their awareness.

If the host is a vegetarian or vegan serving his usual cuisine, you may not be able to low-carb. Think about eating before the event, and then just eat a little to be cordial.

12. REASONABLE EXPECTATIONS

Many people lose three to five pounds (1.4 to 2.3 kg) in the first week or two of the program. If you're one of the lucky ones, enjoy it, brag about it! Tell all your friends about this wonderful Ketogenic Mediterranean Diet! But that rate of loss won't be sustainable or safe for more than a couple weeks. And most of the loss isn't fat. Forget about the grandiose claims of other weight loss plans. If you lose over two pounds (1 kg) per week on my program, averaged over three to four weeks, you're losing too fast and need to eat more. Otherwise you're at risk for medical complications (from nutrient deficiencies) and diet burnout ("I can't stand this anymore. I quit!")

Most people who have reduced their salt intake to help control high blood pressure eventually find they prefer low-salt eating. It may take a couple months. A similar phenomenon happens with Ketogenic Mediterranean eating. It will take at least eight to 12 weeks of practice to alter your preference for your old way of eating. Don't give up early.

I advocate weight loss of about a pound (half a kg) per week, or two pounds (1 kg) at most, mainly because it works over the long run. It's sustainable and safe. The weight lost is indeed fat tissue. Other programs tout losses of three to five pounds per week, but much of that loss is water, muscle protein, or intestinal contents. Your body cannot tolerate this for long and will work against your mind to repair or limit the physiologic damage.

A reasonable rate-of-weight-loss goal also will limit the sense of sacrifice and deprivation that torpedoes so many diets. Even on the KMD, there will be times when you feel deprived of carbohydrates, usually mild and transient. Hey, I never said it was easy! Never forget at those times, when you're most hungry, that's when your body is burning fat. You're instantaneously losing weight.

13. WEIGHT-LOSS STALL

It's common on any weight-loss program to be cruising along losing weight as expected, then suddenly the weight loss stops although you're still far from goal weight. This is the infamous and mysterious stall.

Don't panic. We'll get you through this.

Once you know the reason for the stall, the way to break it becomes obvious. The most common reasons are: 1) you're not really following the full program any more; you've drifted off the path, often unconsciously, 2) instead of eating just until you're full or satisfied, you're stuffing yourself, 3) you need to start or intensify an exercise program (see chapter eight), 4) you've developed an interfering medical problem such as adrenal insufficiency (rare) or an underactive thyroid; see your doctor, 5) you're taking interfering medication such as a steroid; see your doctor, or 6) your strength training program is building new muscle that masks ongoing loss of fat (not a problem!).

If you still can't figure out what's causing your stall, do a nutritional analysis of one weeks' worth of eating, with a focus on daily digestible carb and calorie totals. Resources listed in the Record-Keeping section (No.9) will help with this. You may find you've been sabotaged by "carb creep": excessive dietary carbs have insidiously invaded you.

Even if you're eating very-low-carb, it's still possible to have excess body fat, even gain new fat, if you eat too many calories from protein and fat. It's not easy, but it's possible.

He who enjoys good health is rich, though he knows
it not.

— Italian proverb

The sovereign invigorator of the body is exercise,
and of all the exercises walking is the best.

— Thomas Jefferson

8

A Week of Meals
+ Special Recipes

This chapter provides seven days of meals consistent with the Ketogenic Mediterranean Diet
(KMD). Even if you follow the guidelines and
restrictions "to a T," the KMD provides lots of variety, limited mostly by your imagination. You're going
to eat lots of natural, whole foods made by God, and
few processed, man-made foods.

You don't even have to do any cooking if you don't
want. Avoid cooking altogether by using canned fish
and meats along with raw whole foods and commercially prepared nuts, cheese, olive oil, wine, and
spices. But many will appreciate the added variety
and tastes that cooking brings to the table.

AS SIMPLE AS YOU LIKE

When I was following the KMD myself, a typical day started with a breakfast of cooked eggs with or without bacon, sausage, pre-cooked microwaved bratwurst, or left-over steak or chicken. Lunch was a large salad tossed with both olive oil vinaigrette and canned tuna (or the salad/vinaigrette and a separate tin of sardines or kippered herring). If vinaigrette wasn't at hand, I'd just pour olive oil, vinegar, salt, and pepper into the bowl of salad, then toss. Dinner was another large salad and steak or sautéed chicken and a glass of wine. I ate my daily ounce of nuts whenever I felt like it, and I often had a couple ounces of mozzarella string cheese. If I took my lunch to work, it could be as simple as a can of tuna (eaten with some tartar sauce), an ounce of nuts, and a couple ounces of cheese. Pretty simple if you ask me.

VINAIGRETTES

A homemade vinaigrette is an easy way to get your 2–3 tbsp (30–45 ml) of olive oil daily. The basic recipe is three parts olive oil to one part vinegar. Add salt, pepper, and other spices at your whim. Blend with a whisk, or put all ingredients in a jar with a lid and shake it. Favor red wine or white wine vinegar over balsamic. Balsamic has the highest carb content of the vinegars. I suppose you could use apple cider vinegar, too. See the Special Recipes section of this chapter for a couple fancy vinaigrettes. Mix a batch and keep it in the refrigerator; it should be good for a week. You may be able to find a commercially prepared vinaigrette in the salad dressing section of the supermarket. If so, be sure the oil is predominantly olive oil (not very common) and that a serving (usually 2 tbsp) has no more than 2 g of carb. Vinaigrettes can be used on salads, drizzled on cooked or fresh vegetables, and as marinades for fish, chicken, or beef.

If you're willing to do only minimal cooking, learn how to fry and scramble eggs. For extra credit, learn how to fry or grill steak or chicken, and sauté chicken and vegetables in olive oil.

TIME-SAVING CONVENIENCE

Canned meats and fish are time-savers and often less expensive than fresh, raw products. (Worried about mercury poisoning from fish? I've been practicing medicine for over two decades and haven't seen a case of it yet.) Canned sardines are available with sauces such as tomato, jalapeno, or mustard. Just be sure the sauce doesn't add more than a couple carb grams per 4-ounce (113 g) serving. Also watch out for added carbs in canned meats (chicken, for example). Man-made processed meats such as sausages, Spam, ham, or bacon may have unacceptably high added carbs: if it's got over 2–3 g of carbs per 3 or 4-ounce (85–113 g) serving, take a pass and stick with natural meats.

Canned vegetables are usually OK, too. Consider canned green beans, asparagus, and spinach, for example. These are often criticized for their salt content, but the KMD is naturally low in salt and tends to lower blood pressure, so you don't have to worry about the salt in canned vegetables. Frozen vegetables are also conveniently boiled-in-the-bag or microwaved. (Oh, no . . . that's not cooking, is it?)

Finally, in 2012, the food manufacturers are responding to consumer requests for truly "natural" foods with less man-made ingredients such as high fructose corn syrup (HFCS; pure carbohydrate). Search the shelves of your supermarket and you'll find ketchup and picante sauce without HFCS.

A WEEK OF MENUS

Here are some meal ideas to get you started. Each day's menu conforms fairly well to the Ketogenic Mediterranean Diet. Digestible carb totals for each day are in the 20 to 30 gram range. Average daily calorie count is 1,850, with a range of 1,550 to 1,950. This is more than some will want or need. Just eat until you're full, not stuffed, and save the leftovers for another day. Of the total calories, 8% are from carbohydrate, 65% are from fat, 22% are from protein, and 5% are from alcohol. Calorie contributions from fat and protein vary quite a bit more day-to-day than do calories from carbohydrate.

Regarding olive oil, I tend to prefer extra virgin olive oil over the others. My salt choice is often potassium chloride (e.g., Morton's Lite Salt) rather than sodium chloride (table salt), which may help prevent muscle cramps sometimes seen at the start of very-low-carb eating.

"Dinner" is the evening meal, by the way.

Day 1

Breakfast: Eggs and Bratwurst

3 large eggs
1.5 tbsp (22 ml) olive oil
salt and pepper
1 (66g) pre-cooked bratwurst

144

Sauté eggs in the olive oil, salt and pepper to taste. Microwave a pre-cooked bratwurst. Digestible carb grams: 2.

Lunch: Tossed Tuna Salad and Almonds

3.5 oz (100 g) lettuce
1.5 oz (42 g) chopped onion
5.5 oz (150 g) chunked tomatoes
5-oz can (140 g) of solid white albacore tuna packed
    in water (drain and discard the fluid)
1.5 tbsp (22 ml) extra virgin olive oil
½ tbsp (7.5 ml) balsamic vinegar
salt and pepper
1 oz (28 g) almonds

In a 3-qt (3 liter) bowl, put lettuce, onion, chunked tomatoes, and tuna (3.25 oz or 90 g at this point). Add the olive oil, balsamic vinegar, and salt and pepper to taste. Mix well with a fork. Enjoy almonds separately, before, during, or after salad. Digestible carb grams: 12.

Dinner: Steak and Mushrooms

1.5 tbsp (21 g or 22 ml) butter
2 tsp (10 ml) olive oil
6 oz (170 g) steak
5 oz (140 g) sliced white mushrooms
2 tsp (10 ml) Worcestershire sauce or A.1. Steak
    Sauce
5 oz (150 ml) red wine
salt and pepper

Grill or sauté (with olive oil or butter) the steak. Melt 1.5 tbsp (22 ml) of butter in pan, add mushrooms and cook over medium heat about 3 minutes, stirring frequently. Season steak and mu-

145

shrooms with salt and pepper to taste. Enjoy steak with your favorite steak sauce or Worcestershire sauce, but no more than 2 g of carbs in the sauce (e.g., 2 tsp (10 ml) of A.1. Sauce or Lea & Perrins Worcestershire sauce has 2 g of carb). Digestible carb grams: 10.

Day 2

Breakfast: Mexican Eggs and Avocado

3 large eggs (50 g each)
1 tbsp (14 g or 15 ml) butter
½ cup (240 ml) Pico de Gallo a la Rosa (See Special Recipes at end of this chapter)
1 California avocado (135 g), peeled, seeded, and sliced
salt and pepper

Sauté eggs in butter. Top with ½ cup Pico de Gallo a la Rosa (see Special Recipes). May substitute for Pico de Gallo: any serving of commercial picante sauce with no more than 3 g of digestible carb (digestible carb grams = total carb grams in serving minus fiber grams in serving). Salt and pepper to taste. Digestible carb grams: 7.

Lunch: Tuna Salad Over Lettuce, with Walnuts

1 large egg (50 g)
3 oz (85 g) romaine lettuce
5-oz can of white albacore tuna packed in water (drain and discard the fluid)
½ oz (14 g) onion, diced (about 2 tbsp)
8-inch stalk (40 g or 20-cm stalk) of celery, diced
2 tbsp (30 ml) Miracle Whip Dressing or regular mayonnaise

salt and pepper
dash of lemon (optional)
1 oz (28 g) walnuts

Hard-boil a large egg, then peel and dice. Drain liquid off a 5-ounce can of white albacore tuna (net 3.5 oz or 100 g of fish); empty tuna into bowl. To bowl, add diced egg, diced onion, diced celery, and Miracle Whip Dressing or regular mayonnaise. Mix all together, with salt and pepper and/or a dash of lemon to taste. Place on bed of romaine lettuce. Enjoy walnuts around mealtime. Digestible carb grams: 9.

Dinner: Baked Trout with Snow Peas (sugar snap peas)

7 tbsp (100 g) extra virgin olive oil
5 garlic cloves (15 g), diced
1.5 tbsp (6 g) raw parsley, chopped
1 tsp (5 ml) salt
1 tsp (5 ml) black pepper
¾ fl oz (22 g or ml) lemon juice
4 leaves (1.5 g) fresh basil, chopped
16 oz (450 g) fresh trout
6 oz (170 g) snow peas (sugar snap peas)
5 oz (150 ml) white wine

This recipe provides *two* large servings of fish and *two* servings of snow peas.

In a glass or plastic bowl, mix 5 tbsp (70 g) of the extra virgin olive oil, 3 of the diced garlic cloves (9 g), the chopped raw parsley, salt, black pepper, the lemon juice, and the chopped basil. This is your marinade.

Place fresh trout filets in a medium sized (8–9" or 20–23 cm diameter) glass baking dish, then cover with marinade. Let sit in refrigerator for 1–2 hours, turning occasionally. Preheat oven to 375°F (190°C). Pull fish dish out of refrigerator once you start the preheat process. Cover glass dish with aluminum foil, then bake in oven for 20–40 minutes. Cooking time depends on your oven and the thickness of the fish. Thin filets about 1/2" (1.25 cm) thick may be done in 20–25 minutes. Thicker fish (1" or 2.5 cm)) may take 30–45 minutes. This is a judgment call. When done, it should flake apart readily with a fork. This works well for trout, salmon, cod, tilapia, and perhaps others. Consider squeezing fresh lemon juice on cooked fish for extra zing.

Now the snow peas. Snap off and discard both tips of the snow pea pods. Sauté 2 diced garlic cloves (6 g) in olive oil over medium heat until soft, perhaps a couple minutes. To the pan add the snow peas. Salt and pepper to taste. Stir snow peas often, if not continuously, while cooking over medium heat, about 3 minutes. Enjoy 5 oz (150 ml) white wine with your meal. Digestible carb grams in wine and half the fish, half the snow peas: 11.

Day 3

Breakfast: Bacon and Eggs

3 large eggs (50 g each)
1.5 tbsp (22 ml) olive oil
6 slices pork bacon, cured (about 50 g cooked)

Fry the eggs in olive oil. Bake or fry the bacon. Digestible carb grams: 2.

Lunch: Chicken Salad Over Mixed Greens

1 large egg (50 g)
4 oz (110 g) cooked, diced chicken (canned or
    freshly sautéed in olive oil)
½ oz (14 g) raw onion, diced (about 2 tbsp)
8-inch stalk (40 g or 20-cm stalk) of raw celery,
    diced
2.5 tbsp (40 ml) Miracle Whip Dressing or regular
    Mayonnaise
2 oz (60 g) romaine lettuce
2 oz (60 g) raw baby spinach
1 oz (28 g) almonds
salt and pepper

Hard-boil an egg, then peel and dice. In a bowl,
place the chicken and add the egg, onion, celery,
and Miracle Whip Dressing or regular mayonnaise.
Mix all together, with salt and pepper and/or a dash
of lemon juice to taste. Place on bed of lettuce and
baby spinach. Enjoy almonds around mealtime or
later as a snack. Digestible carb grams: 10.

Dinner: Baked Balsamic Salmon and Green Beans

16 oz (450 g) salmon filets
salt and pepper
4 cloves (12 g) garlic, minced
1 tbsp (15 ml) olive oil
1.5 oz (45 ml) white wine for the glaze
4.5 tsp (22 ml) mustard
4 tbsp (60 ml) balsamic vinegar
1 tbsp (15 ml) granulated Splenda (or 1 packet (1g)
    of tabletop Splenda)
1.5 tbsp (22 ml) fresh chopped oregano (or 1 tsp
    (5 ml) dried oregano)
7 oz (200 g) canned green beans (or fresh green
    beans sautéed in olive oil/garlic)
5 oz (150 ml) dry white wine

This makes two large servings.

Preheat oven to 400°F (200°C). Line a baking sheet or pan (8" or 20 cm) with aluminum foil. Lightly salt and pepper the fish in the lined pan, with the skin side down.

Now the glaze. Sauté the minced garlic in olive oil in a small saucepan over medium heat for about three minutes, until it's soft. Then add and mix white wine (1.5 oz), mustard, vinegar, granulated Splenda, and 1/8 tsp (0.625 ml) salt. Simmer uncovered over low or medium heat until slightly thickened, about three minutes. Remove glaze from heat and spoon about half of it into a separate container for later use.

Drizzle and brush the salmon in the pan with the glaze left in the saucepan. Sprinkle the oregano on top.

Bake the fish in the oven for about 10–13 minutes, or until it flakes easily with a fork. Cooking time depends on your oven and thickness of the fish. Overcooking the fish will toughen it and dry it out. When done, use a turner to transfer the fish to plates, leaving the skin on the foil if able. Drizzle the glaze from the separate container over the filets with a spoon, or brush it on. Don't use the unwashed brush you used earlier on the raw fish.

Heat canned green beans (7 oz or 200 g) on stovetop or serve at room temperature straight out of the can.

Enjoy a 5-oz glass of dry white wine with your meal. This recipe makes two servings of fish and green beans. Digestible carb grams in wine, half the fish, half the green beans: 14.

[The *balsamic* vinegar adds six g of carb to each serving. To reduce vinegar carbs to zero, you could try this recipe with red wine vinegar, white wine vinegar, or cider vinegar. I've not tried that. Digestible carbs per serving would drop to 8 g.]

Day 4

Breakfast: Steak and Avocado

4 oz (110 g) raw steak
1 California avocado, peeled, seeded, and sliced
    (136 g)
½ tbsp (7 ml) olive oil (optional)
salt and pepper
1 tbsp (15 ml) vinaigrette (see Special Recipes) or
    commercial Italian dressing (regular, not low-fat,
    with less than 2 g of carb per tbsp or 15 ml)

Cook the steak over medium heat, adding half a tbsp (7 ml) olive oil at the start if desired. Salt and pepper to taste. Peel and slice an avocado. Dress avocado with homemade vinaigrette (see Special Recipes) or commercial Italian dressing. Salt and pepper to taste. Digestible carb grams: 4.

Lunch: Avocado Cucumber Salad

5 oz (140 g) cucumber, peeled and sliced into
    rounds
1 California avocado, peeled, seeded, and sliced
    (136 g)
2 tbsp (30 ml) AMD vinaigrette (see Special Recipes)
    or commercial Italian dressing described below

salt and pepper
dash of lime or lemon juice (optional)
1 oz walnuts

Mix the cucumber and avocado in a bowl with the
AMD vinaigrette or commercial Italian dressing
(regular, not low-fat, with 3 g or fewer carbs per 2
tbsp or 30 ml). Salt and pepper to taste. For extra
zing, add a dash of lemon or lime juice. Enjoy the
walnuts on the side now, or mid-afternoon as a
snack. Digestible carb grams: 10.

Dinner: Bacon Shrimp Salad

2 slices (15 g) pork bacon, cured, cooked (or
    substitute 2 tbsp (30 ml) commercial real bacon
    bits)
2 tbsp (30 ml) AMD vinaigrette (see Special Recipes)
    or commercial Italian dressing as below
½ packet of tabletop Splenda
4 oz (110 g) fresh baby spinach
4 oz (110 g) cooked shrimp (Consider commercial
    pre-cooked, peeled shrimp to save time.)
6 oz (180 ml) dry white wine

Cook two bacon slices over medium heat, then
crumble or cut in to tiny pieces (or substitute commercial real bacon bits). Add a half packet of Splenda to the AMD vinaigrette or commercial Italian
dressing (regular, not low-fat, with 3 g or fewer
carbs per 2 tbsp or 30 ml), then mix. On a bed of
fresh baby spinach, place cooked shrimp, then top
with bacon pieces and vinaigrette. Enjoy with 6 oz
dry white wine. Digestible carb grams: 9.

Day 5

Breakfast: Mexican Scrambled Eggs

4 large eggs (50 g each)
1.5 tbsp (22 ml) olive oil
4 tbsp (60 ml) Pico de Gallo a la Rose (see Special
    Recipes) or commercial picante sauce (having 2 g
    or fewer carbs per 2 tbsp)
salt and pepper

Whisk the eggs until smooth, add salt and pepper to taste; set aside. Heat the olive oil in a medium-sized frying pan then add the eggs and cook until done, scrambling now and then. Transfer to plate and top with 4 tbsp (60 ml) Pico de Gallo a al Rosa. Digestible carb grams: 6.

Lunch: Low-Carb Chili

1 cup (240 ml) Low-Carb Chili (see Special Recipes)
1 oz (28 g) almonds

Enjoy 1 oz of almonds around mealtime or later as a snack. Digestible carb grams: 13.

Dinner: Shark and Broccoli

4 oz (110 g) shark, raw
2 cloves (3 g) garlic, peeled and diced
3 tbsp (45 ml) olive oil
1.5 cups (150 g) chopped raw broccoli
salt and pepper
6 oz (180 ml) dry white wine

Lightly salt and pepper the shark, then set aside. Sauté the garlic in 2 tbsp (30 cc) of the olive oil a few minutes over medium heat. Then add the broccoli and sauté to your preference, adding salt and pepper to taste. Remove to a dish. Add another 1 tbsp (15 ml) olive oil to the pan and sauté the shark at medium heat until done, careful not to overcook. Enjoy with dry white wine. Digestible carb grams: 11.

Day 6

Breakfast: Chicken Salad Over Greens

1 large egg (50 g)
5-oz can (150 g) of cooked chicken (drain and
    discard liquid)
½ oz (14 g) onion (2 tbsp or 30 ml), diced
½ stick (40 g) of celery, diced
2 tbsp (30 ml) Miracle Whip Salad Dressing or
    Regular mayonnaise (not low-fat)
salt and pepper
2 oz (60 g) romaine lettuce
2 oz (60 g) raw baby spinach
dash of lemon or lime juice (optional)
1 oz (28 g) walnuts

Hard-boil the large egg, then peel and dice. Place the chicken into a bowl then add the egg, diced onion, diced celery, and the Miracle Whip Salad Dressing. Mix all together, with salt and pepper and/or a dash of lemon or lime juice to taste. Place on bed of romaine lettuce and fresh baby spinach. Enjoy walnuts around mealtime or later as a snack. Digestible carb grams: 11.

Lunch: Kippered Herring and Cheese

3.5 oz (100 g) canned kippered herring
3 oz (80 g) cheese

Digestible carb grams: 2.

Dinner: Hamburger and Salad

8 oz (225 g) raw hamburger meat
1 oz (28 g) onion, finely chopped
1 tbsp (15 ml) A.1. Steak Sauce or Worcestershire
    sauce
salt and pepper
3 oz (85 g) lettuce
3 oz (85 g) tomato, cut into chunks
2 oz (60 g) cucumber, peeled and sliced
1.5 tbsp (22 ml) olive oil
½ tbsp (7 ml) vinegar

To the raw hamburger meat, add the chopped
onion, A.1. Steak Sauce or Worcestershire sauce,
and salt and pepper to taste. Blend thoroughly with
your hands. (No particular need for *lean* hamburger;
it's your choice.) Cook in pan over medium heat.
While cooking, prepare your salad.

In a bowl, place the lettuce, tomato chunks, sliced
cucumber, and finally, the olive oil and vinegar. Mix
salad thoroughly. Salt and pepper to taste.

Enjoy with 6 oz of red wine. Digestible carb grams:
13.

Day 7

Breakfast: Brats and Tomatoes

6 oz (170 g) tomato, sliced
2 tbsp (30 ml) AMD vinaigrette (see Special Recipes)
    or commercial Italian dressing (regular, not
    low-fat, with 3 g or fewer carbs per 2 tbsp or
    30 ml)
salt and pepper
2 pre-cooked bratwursts (about 2.3 oz or 65 g each)
6 tsp (30 ml) mustard (optional)

Dress the tomato slices with the vinaigrette, plus
salt and pepper to taste. Heat 2 pre-cooked bratwursts as instructed on package. Use mustard on
the brats if desired. Digestible carb grams: 8.

Lunch: Easy Tuna Plus Pecans

5-oz can (140 g) of albacore tuna
2 tbsp (30 ml) Miracle Whip Salad Dressing (or real,
    high-fat mayonnaise)
1 tsp (5 ml) lemon or lime juice
1 oz (28 g) pecan halves

Drain the liquid off the can of tuna then place tuna
in a bowl. Add Miracle Whip Salad Dressing and
lemon or lime juice. Mix thoroughly and enjoy. Eat
1 oz of pecan halves around mealtime or later as a
snack. If you want to simplify this, forget the Miracle Whip and lemon; just use 1 oz (28 g) of commercial tartar sauce that derives at least 80% of
calories from fat and has less than 3 g of carb per 2
tbsp or 30 ml. Digestible carb grams: 5.

Dinner: Ham Salad

2 oz (60 g) cooked ham, cut in to small cubes
1 oz (28 g) celery, sliced and diced
1 oz (28 g) seedless grapes (about 4 grapes), cut into small chunks
1 oz (28 g) walnuts, coarsely crumbled
4 oz (110 g) romaine lettuce
3 tbsp AMD vinaigrette or commercial Italian,
    French, or ranch dressing having 2 or fewer
    grams of carb per 2 tbsp or 30 ml)

Lay out a bed of lettuce then sprinkle these on top: ham, celery, grapes, walnuts. Finish construction with AMD vinaigrette or commercial dressing. You're done. Alternatively, substitute cooked chicken or steak for ham. With chicken, apple may work better than grapes. If having a glass of wine (6 fl oz or 180 ml) with meal, delete the grapes or the carb count will be too high. Digestible carb grams: 10.

(When commercial dressing is used, the digestible carb count is closer to 13 than 10 g.)

SPECIAL RECIPES

Nutrient analysis of these recipes is compliments of SELF-NutritionData. You can analyze your own recipes there, finding the amounts of 40+ nutrients. The web address is http://nutritiondata.self.com/.

ARIZONA'S BAKED CHEESECAKE

My daughter, Arizona, enjoys baking. I'm nudging her into low-carb baking since I miss my sweets.

Arizona usually prepares the commercial cheesecakes based on a pre-mixed box: you add some

KMD

fresh ingredients, mix, then refrigerate. The baked cheesecake here is more work, but I think well worth the effort. We had fun making this together.

Ingredients for crust:

1.5 cups (226 g) ground nuts (pecan, walnut, or almond)
5.5 tbsp (82 ml) melted butter
½ tsp (2 g) ground cinnamon
1 egg white (33 g)
1 tbsp (15 ml) Granulated Splenda No Calorie Sweetener (optional)

Ingredients for filling:

24 oz (675 g) cream cheese
1 cup (230 g) sour cream
4 large eggs (50 g each)
1 cup (28 g) Granulated Splenda No Calorie Sweetener
juice from one lemon (47 g or ml)
2 tsp (10 ml) vanilla extract

Preparation

Have the following ingredients at room temperature before you start: eggs, cream cheese, sour cream.

Preheat oven to 350°F (175°C).

First, the crust. Put ground pecans, 4 tbsp (60 ml) of the melted butter (fine to microwave briefly), cinnamon, granulated Splenda, and egg white in bowl, then blend all. Spread onto bottom of greased (with melted butter, the last 1.5 tbsp or 22 ml) 9" (20–25 cm) springform pan. Cover with plastic wrap to aid spreading evenly; remove and discard plastic wrap after spreading the crust. Bake in 350°F (175°C) oven for 10–15 minutes then remove. Then reduce heat to 325°F (160°C).

Filling: Use a mixer on low to medium setting to beat the cream cheese until fluffy. Blend in the Splenda incrementally, a little at a time, beating until creamy. Then mix in the lemon juice and vanilla extract. Gently mix in one egg at a time and beat on low speed after each egg. Mix in the sour cream last. Pour cream cheese mixture into the crusted spring-form pan. Place on the top rack in the 325°F (160°C) preheated oven for 50–60 minutes. On the rack below that, place a pie pan full of water. [The water pan and gentle handling of the eggs help prevent cracking of the final product.] When time is up, turn off the oven and open the oven door but leave the cake in the oven to cool slowly. After an hour, remove from oven. After it cools to room temperature, put it in the refrigerator to age for 24 hours.

Notes:

■ The filling has one cup of Splenda, which I estimate is one ounce (28 g). This has 96 calories, which I assume is mostly from maltodextrin rather than sucralose.
■ Many cooks just use a glass pie pan instead of the springform pan. The volume of this recipe is likely too much for a 9″ (23 cm) pie pan, so you could reduce the amounts; or make a larger pie or two smaller ones.
■ Some cooks don't bother to bake the crust first.
■ Reduce the carb count even further by omitting the crust.
■ For higher fiber, substitute flax meal for about a third or ½ of the ground nuts.
■ The Splenda in this recipe is not the same as in the individual serving packets.

KMD

Nutrient analysis:

Recipe makes 12 servings. Each serving has 444 calories, 8 g carbohydrate, 2 g fiber, 6 g digestible carbohydrate, 8 g protein, 43 g fat. 6% of calories are from carbohydrate, 8% from protein, 86% from fat.

LOW-CARB CHILI

It's spicy, but not hot spicy. Peeled and sliced cold cucumbers make a nice side dish. If your children or housemates aren't eating low-carb, they may enjoy the chili mixed 50:50 with cheese macaroni, and buttered cornbread on the side.

Ingredients

20 oz (567 g) raw ground beef, 80% lean meat/20% fat
20 oz (567 g) raw pork Italian sausage
1 large onion
14.5 oz (411 g) canned diced tomatoes
4 oz (113 g) tomato paste
1 tbsp (15 ml) dry unsweetened cocoa powder
5 garlic cloves
½ tsp (2.5 ml) salt
¼ tsp (1.2 ml) ground allspice
2 tbsp (30 ml) chili powder
¼ tsp (1.2 ml) ground cinnamon
½ tbsp (7.5 ml) ground cumin
¼ tsp (1.2 ml) ground cayenne pepper
2 packets (1 g per packet) Splenda tabletop sweetener
1 cup (240 ml) water

Preparation

Cut the Italian sausage into small pieces. Sauté the sausage, ground beef, onions, and garlic in a large pot. Don't just brown the meat, cook it thoroughly. When done, drain off the fat if desired. Add the remainder of ingredients, bring to a boil, then simmer for about an hour. Add additional water if the chili looks too thick. Makes eight cups. Serving size is one cup (240 ml).

Nutrient Analysis:

Recipe makes 8 servings of 1 cup (240 ml). Each serving has 492 calories, 14 g carbohydrate, 3 g fiber, 11 g digestible carbohydrate, 24 g protein, 38 g fat. 10% of calories are from carbohydrate, 21% from protein, 69% from fat.

Notes: Analysis is based on fat not being drained from the cooked meat. Calorie count and calories from fat would be a bit lower if you drained off fat.

PICO DE GALLO A LA ROSA

Try this, for example, over fried eggs.

Ingredients

6 oz (170 g) tomatoes
2 oz (56 g) onion
1 jalapeno pepper (14 g)
3–4 tbsp (2 g) cilantro
salt

Preparation

Chop all vegetables very finely. Use the entire jalapeno, including seeds, but not the stem. If you prefer less spicy heat, use less jalapeno and discard the
seeds. Combine all ingredients after chopping. Salt
to taste. Eat at room temperature, chilled, or heated
at medium heat in a saucepan (about 5 minutes,
until jalapenos lose their intense green color).
Makes 1.25 cups.

Nutrient Analysis:

Recipe makes about three servings of ½ cup (120
ml) each. One serving has 80 calories, 4 g carb, 1 g
fiber, 3 g digestible carb, 1 g protein, minimal fat.
83% of calories are from carbohydrate, 10% from
protein, 7% from fat.

ALMOND POUND CAKE

My son, Paul, and I had a great time making this
when he was 11-years-old, around the time he an-
nounced he "might be interested in a career as a
culinary professional." This cake was our first joint
baking project.

2 cups (224 g) almond flour
½ cup (113 g) butter at room temperature
4 oz (116 g) cream cheese at room temperature
1 cup (28 g) Splenda Granulated No Calorie Swee-
    tener
6 eggs, medium size (44 g each), at room tempera-
    ture
1 tsp (5 ml) baking powder
1 tbsp (15 ml) lemon zest (or 1.5 tsp or 7 ml lemon
    extract)
1 tsp (5 ml) vanilla extract

If you can't find almond flour, make your own by grinding almonds into the consistency of a flour. You can do this in a blender or electric coffee bean grinder.

Preparation

Preheat oven to 350°F (175°C).

Mix the butter, cream cheese, and Splenda with a hand-held or table-top mixer, then beat in the eggs one at a time, mixing thoroughly after each egg. In a separate container, mix the baking powder into the almond flour. Add the almond flour a little at a time into the butter/sour cream bowl, beating as you go. Then mix in vanilla extract and lemon zest. Pour into a 9-inch (22-24 cm) cake pan greased with butter, vegetable oil, or Baker's Joy Baking Spray, then bake at 350°F (175°C). for 35-40 minutes.

Nutrient Analysis:

Recipe makes 12 servings. Each serving has 248 calories, 5 g carbohydrate, 1 g fiber, 4 g digestible carbohydrate, 5 g protein, 18 g fat. 27% of calories are from carbohydrate, 9% from protein, 64% from fat.

AMD VINAIGRETTE

Try this on salads, fresh vegetables, or as a marinade for chicken, fish, or beef. If using as a marinade, keep the entree/marinade combo in the refrigerator for 4–24 hours. Seasoned vinaigrettes taste even better if you let them sit for several hours after preparation. This recipe was in my first book, *The Advanced Mediterranean Diet*; hence, "AMD vinaigrette."

Ingredients

1 clove (3 g) garlic
juice from ½ lemon (23 g or ml)
a third of a cup (78 ml) oil olive
2 tbsp (8 g) fresh parsley
½ tsp (2.5 ml)) salt
½ tsp (2.5 ml) yellow mustard
½ tsp (1.2 ml) paprika
2 tbsp (30 ml) vinegar, red wine,

Preparation

In a bowl, combine all ingredients and whisk together. Alternatively, you can put all ingredients in a jar with a lid and shake vigorously. Let sit at room temperature for an hour, for flavors to meld. Then refrigerate. It should "keep" for at least 5 days in refrigerator. Shake before using. Servings per batch: 3.

Nutrient Analysis:

Recipe makes 3 servings (2 tbsp or 30 ml per serving). Each serving has 220 calories, 2 g digestible carb, almost no fiber, negligible protein, 24 g fat. 3% of calories are from carbohydrate, 97% from fat.

MUSTARD VINAIGRETTE

Try this on salads, fresh vegetables, or as a marinade for chicken, fish, or beef. If using as a marinade, keep the entree/marinade combo in the refrigerator for 4–24 hours.

Ingredients

3 tsp (15 ml) yellow mustard, yellow
¾ cup (177 ml) olive oil
½ tsp (2.5 ml) salt
½ tsp (2.5 ml) pepper (fresh ground if available)
¼ cup (60 ml) cider vinegar

Preparation

Mix all ingredients in a jar with a lid. Shake vigorously to create an emulsion. Let sit at room temperature for an hour, for flavors to meld. Then refrigerate. Should "keep" for at least 5 days in refrigerator. Shake before using. Makes one cup.

Nutrient Analysis:

Recipe makes one cup (8 servings of 2 tbsp each).
Each serving has 182 calories, negligible carbs, zero
protein, 20 g fat. 1% of calories are from carbohydrate, 99% from fat.

White flour is better suited to glue for kindergarten art projects than to nutrition.

> —Drs. Eric Westman, Stephen Phinney, and
> Jeff Volek in *The New Atkins for a New You*

9

WHAT? ME EXERCISE?

"Aunt Cheryl, would you take us to Sea World? Please, please, please, please, please?!"

Cheryl was babysitting her eight and 10 year old nieces while their parents were away for the weekend celebrating their wedding anniversary. She stalled for time while trying to come up with an alternative. The kids were bouncing off the walls with energy. Cheryl had enjoyed Sea World 10 years ago, but also remembered the size of the park and how much walking was involved between Shamu and the seal show, and all the exhibits in between.

She was 80 pounds (36 kg) heavier now and knew she couldn't hack it. She fantasized about the kids bolting ahead of her and getting lost in the crowd. What would she tell her brother? "Your daughters were kidnapped because I'm so fat. Sorry."

Mustering all her enthusiasm, she told the children, "Hey! I've got a better idea. Let's go to Chuckie Cheese's instead!" She could safely turn the girls loose there while she sat in a booth reading, eating pizza, and drinking a diet Coke. The girls acquiesced, and off they went. Cheryl wondered if they remembered her huffing, puffing, and sweating her way around the city zoo two years ago.

Shopping at the mall was Cheryl's favorite form of exercise. Uncommonly generous, Cheryl was famous among her friends and relatives for surprising them with unexpected thoughtful tchotchkes as well as more substantial gifts. Walking in from the mall parking lot plus two hours strolling about was a decent workout. But she did it only every couple weeks. For three hours a week, she volunteered to deliver Meals-On-Wheels, carrying meals into houses and apartments. She spent much more time driving than walking. Of course, she wasn't doing it for the exercise.

Cheryl's only other regular physical activities were housework and walking to and from the parking lot at her job as a librarian. She had hated PE class in school. She never understood why someone would want to exercise when they could spend that time reading, playing cards, relaxing with TV, or playing piano.

By the time she finished gaining those 80 excess pounds (36 kg) of fat between the ages of 20 and 30, she was feeling tired all the time. Her stamina was kaput. She knew 60-year-olds who had more energy than she did. Her knees were aching after the mall trips. She was too young to feel this way! Was there something going on physically other than being overweight? Perhaps diabetes, Chronic Fatigue Syndrome, or a hidden cancer? Most of her relatives were heavy and few of them lived beyond age 65, succumbing to strokes or various cancers. Several relatives had diabetes.

Cheryl's favorite aunt died of cancer at the age of 56. Cheryl, in her early 30s, came to see me six weeks after the funeral. "Doctor Parker, why do I feel so old and tired?" A thorough physical exam and diagnostic lab work revealed only early knee arthritis, mildly elevated blood pressure, and obesity (220 pounds or 100 kg). I was certain that losing the excess weight plus an increase in physical activity would help her immensely. I knew also that convincing her, much less altering her behavior, would be an uphill battle. But I was prepared to help her win it.

EXERCISE AND WEIGHT LOSS

Have you seen TV's "Biggest Loser" show? Contestants do lose a huge amount of weight through a combination of extreme amounts of exercise (several hours daily) and major calorie restriction. Participants are pulled out of their usual living situation and put in a supportive yet highly competitive environment. They're competing for their 15 minutes of TV fame, as well as substantial money: $250,000 in the U.S. version. If you can replicate that setting, exercise does indeed help with weight loss. But that's an unrealistic scenario for most of us.

Exercise is overrated as a pathway to major weight loss. For the average person wanting to lose excess weight, regular exercise may contribute about 10% to a successful effort, with the other 90% coming from the eating end of the equation.

If you know from past experience that exercise helps you lose weight, then work it.

On the other hand, what's the role of exercise in *maintenance of weight loss*? In other words, does exercise help prevent weight regain? Yes. Surveys of successful long-term "losers" consistently show that regular exercise is strongly linked to prevention of regain. We're looking at 45 to 60 minutes of exercise on most days of the week.

If you're going to invest that much of your time, you'll be glad to know that regular physical activity has lots of other beneficial effects.

EXERCISE BENEFITS

DEATH PREVENTION AND POSTPONEMENT

As many as 250,000 deaths per year in the United States (approximately 12% of the total) are attributable to a lack of regular physical activity. We know now that regular physical activity can prevent a significant number of these deaths. Exercise induces metabolic changes that lessen the impact of, or prevent altogether, several major illnesses, such as high blood pressure, coronary artery disease, diabetes, and obesity.

PHYISCAL FITNESS AND AEROBIC POWER

To understand how exercise prevents and postpones death, we need to first define exercise, physical fitness, and aerobic power.

Exercise is planned, structured, and repetitive bodily movement done to improve or maintain physical fitness.

Physical fitness is a set of attributes that relate to your ability to perform physical activity. These attributes include resting heart rate, blood pressure at rest and during exercise, lung capacity, body composition (weight in relation to height, percentage of body fat and muscle, bone structure), and aerobic power.

Aerobic power takes some explanation. Muscles perform their work by contracting, which shortens the muscles, pulling on attached tendons or bones. The resultant movement is physical activity. Muscle contraction requires energy, which is obtained from chemical reactions that use oxygen. Oxygen from the air we breathe is delivered to muscle tissue by the lungs, heart, and blood vessels. The ability of the cardiopulmonary system to transport oxygen from the atmosphere to the working muscles is called maximal oxygen uptake, or aerobic power. It's the primary factor limiting performance of muscular activity.

Aerobic power is commonly measured by having a person perform progressively more difficult exercise on a treadmill or bicycle to the point of exhaustion. The treadmill test starts at a walking pace and gets faster and steeper every few minutes. The longer the subject can last on the treadmill, the greater his aerobic power. A large aerobic power is one of the most reliable indicators of good physical fitness. It's cultivated through consistent, repetitive physical activity.

Higher levels of physical fitness are linked to lower rates of death primarily from cancer and cardiovascular disease (e.g., heart attacks and stroke). What's more, moving from a lower to a higher level of fitness also prolongs life, even for people over 60. How do you get from a lower to higher level of fitness? Start an exercise program or intensify an existing one.

METABOLIC EFFECTS OF EXERCISE

Where does the fat go when you lose weight dieting? Chemical reactions convert it to energy, water, and carbon dioxide, which weigh less than the fat. In terms of losing weight, an important metabolic effect of exercise is that it turns fat into weightless energy.

Furthermore, exercise counteracts the decrease in basal metabolic rate seen with some calorie-restricted diets. In some folks, exercise temporarily reduces appetite (but others note the opposite effect). While caloric restriction during dieting can diminish your sense of energy and vitality, exercise typically does the opposite. Many dieters, especially those on low-calorie poorly designed diets, lose lean tissue (such as muscle and water) in addition to fat. This isn't desirable over the long run. Exercise counteracts the tendency to lose muscle mass while nevertheless modestly facilitating fat loss.

FOUNTAIN OF YOUTH

Regular exercise is a demonstrable "fountain of youth." Peak aerobic power (or fitness) naturally diminishes by 50% between young adulthood and age 65. In other words, as age advances even a light physical task becomes fatiguing if it is sustained over time. By the age of 75 or 80, many of us depend on others for help with the ordinary tasks of daily living, such as housecleaning and grocery shopping. Regular exercise increases fitness (aerobic power) by 15–20% in middle-aged and older men and women, the equivalent of a 10–20 year reduction in biological age! This prolongation of self-sufficiency improves quality of life.

HEART HEALTH

Exercise helps control multiple cardiac (heart attack) risk factors: obesity, high cholesterol, elevated blood pressure, high triglycerides, and diabetes.

Regular aerobic activity tends to lower LDL cholesterol, the "bad cholesterol." Jogging 10 or 12 miles a week, or the equivalent amount of other exercise, increases HDL cholesterol ("good cholesterol") substantially.

Exercise increases heart muscle efficiency and blood flow to the heart. For the person who has already had a heart attack, regular physical activity decreases the incidence of fatal recurrence by 20–30% and adds an extra two or three years of life, on average.

EFFECT ON DIABETES

Eighty-five percent of type 2 diabetics are overweight or obese. It's not just a random association. Obesity contributes heavily to most cases of type 2 diabetes, particularly in those predisposed by heredity. Insulin is the key that allows bloodstream sugar (glucose) into cells for utilization as energy, thus keeping blood sugar from reaching dangerously high levels. Overweight bodies produce plenty of insulin, often more than average. The problem in overweight diabetics is that the cells are no longer sensitive to insulin's effect. Weight loss and exercise independently return insulin sensitivity towards normal. Many diabetics can improve their condition through sensible exercise and weight management.

173

MISCELLANEOUS BENEFITS

In case you need more reasons to start or keep exercising, consider the following additional benefits: 1) enhanced immune function, 2) stronger bones, 3) preservation and improvement of flexibility, 4) diminished premenstrual bloating, breast tenderness, and mood changes, 5) reduced incidence of dementia, 6) less trouble with constipation, 7) better ability to handle stress, 8) less trouble with insomnia, 9) improved self-esteem, 10) enhanced sense of well-being, with less anxiety and depression, 11) higher perceived level of energy, and 12) prevention of weight regain.

EXERCISE RECOMMENDATIONS

Now that you know the health benefits of exercise, it's a little easier to understand those crazy people you see jogging at 6 a.m. in below-freezing weather. I'm sure you're ready to join them tomorrow morning. Right? Wait . . . what?

Here's some good news. Most people following the Ketogenic Mediterranean Diets are able to lose excess weight without starting an exercise program. Many, but certainly not all, will be able to maintain a stable, reasonable weight long-term without ongoing exercise. However, for the reasons already outlined, I recommend you start a physical activity program eventually.

I must warn you that athletic individuals who perform vigorous exercise should expect a deterioration in performance levels during the first three to four weeks of any very-low-carb ketogenic diet, including the Ketogenic Mediterranean Diet. The body needs that time to adjust to burning mostly fat for fuel rather than carbohydrate.

Also, competitive weight-lifters or other anaerobic athletes (e.g., sprinters) may be hampered by the low muscle glycogen stores that accompany ketogenic diets. They need more carbohydrates for high-level performance.

HOW MUCH EXERCISE?

All I'm asking you to do, eventually, is aerobic activity, such as walk briskly (3–4 mph or 4.8–6.4 km/h) for 30 minutes most days of the week, and do some muscle-strengthening exercises three times a week. This amount of exercise will get you most of the documented health benefits. It's OK if you want to wait until you've lost some of your excess weight, but I probably wouldn't.

Keep reading to find out if exercise would be a bad idea for you

The U.S. Centers for Disease Control and Prevention recommends at least 150 minutes per week of moderate-intensity aerobic activity (e.g., brisk walking) and muscle-strengthening activity at least twice a week, OR 75 minutes per week of vigorous-intensity aerobic activity (e.g., running or jogging) plus muscle-strengthening activity at least twice a week. The muscle-strengthening activity should work all the major muscle groups: legs, hips, back, abdomen, chest, shoulders, arms.

Please note that you don't have to run marathons (26.2 miles or 42.2 km) or compete in the Ironman Triathlon to earn the health benefits of exercise.

175

However, if health promotion and disease prevention are your goals, plan on a lifetime commitment to regular physical activity.

Don't feel bad if you haven't been exercising; you're not alone. Twenty-five percent of U.S. adults are completely sedentary. Only two or three of every 10 Americans are active enough to gain all the health benefits of exercise.

STRENGTH TRAINING

What's "strength training"? It's also called muscle-strengthening activity, resistance training, weight training, and resistance exercise. Examples include lifting weights, work with resistance bands, digging, shoveling, yoga, push-ups, chin-ups, and other exercises that use your body weight or other loads for resistance.

Strength training three times a week increases your strength and endurance, allows you to sculpt your body to an extent, and counteracts the loss of lean body mass (muscle) so often seen during efforts to lose excess weight. It also helps maintain your functional abilities as you age. For example, it's a major chore for many 80-year-olds to climb a flight of stairs, carry in a bag of groceries from the car, or vacuum a house. Strength training helps maintain these abilities that youngsters take for granted.

According to the U.S. Centers for Disease Control and Prevention: "To gain health benefits, muscle-strengthening activities need to be done to the point where it's hard for you to do another repetition without help. A repetition is one complete movement of an activity, like lifting a weight or doing a sit-up. Try to do 8–12 repetitions per activity that count as 1 set. Try to do at least 1 set of muscle-strengthening activities, but to gain even more benefits, do 2 or 3 sets."

If this is starting to sound like Greek to you, consider instruction by a personal trainer at a local gym or health club. That's a good investment for anyone unfamiliar with strength training in view of its great benefits. You can waste much time and easily hurt yourself if you do it wrong. Alternatives to a personal trainer would be help from an experienced friend or instructional DVD. If you're determined to go it alone, Internet resources may help, but be careful. Consider "Growing Stronger: Strength Training for Older Adults" (http://www.cdc.gov/physicalactivity/downloads/growing_stronger.pdf). Doug Robb's blog, HealthHabits, is a wonderful source of strength training advice (http://www.healthhabits.ca/).

In 2011, I made a serious commitment to Mark Verstegen's Core Performance workout program. Done in the privacy of my home, it combines strength training, cardio (aerobics), flexibility, and balance training. I'm very happy with results. Check out his book at Amazon.com.

Current strength training techniques are much different than what you remember from high school 30 years ago. Modern methods are better. Some of the latest research suggests that strength training may be even more beneficial than aerobic exercise.

AEROBIC ACTIVITY

What's "aerobic activity"? Just about anything that mostly makes you huff and puff. In other words, get short of breath to some degree. It's also called "cardio." Examples are brisk walking, swimming, golf (pulling a cart or carrying clubs), lawn work, painting, home repair, racket sports and table tennis, house cleaning, leisurely canoeing, jogging, bicycling, jumping rope, and skiing. The possibilities are endless. A leisurely stroll in the shopping mall doesn't qualify, unless that makes you short of breath. Don't laugh: that *is* a workout for many who are obese.

But which aerobic physical activity is best? Glad you asked!

The most important criterion is that it be pleasant for you. If not outright fun, it should be often enjoyable and always tolerable.

Your exercise of choice should also be available year-round, affordable, safe, and utilize large muscle groups. The greater mass and number of muscles used, the more calories you will burn, which is important if you're trying to lose weight or prevent gain. Your largest muscles are in your legs, so consider walking, biking, team sports, ski machines, jogging, treadmill, swimming, water aerobics, stationary cycling, stair-steppers, tennis, volleyball, roller-skating, rowing, jumping rope, and yard work.

The following table lists the average number of calories burned during a few types of aerobic physical activity for a person weighing 150 pounds (68 kg). Heavier people would tend to expend more calories. Calories burned during your particular physical activity are difficult to predict and measure. But don't choose an activity just because it burns lots of calories. That's a certain path to injury or quick burn out. Then you won't be exercising at all.

Calories Expended by a 150-Pound (68 kg) Person
in 15 Minutes of Various Activities

Activity	Calories
Walking 2 mph (3.2 km/h)	60
Walking 3 mph (4.8 km/h)	75
Walking 4 mph (6.4 km/h)	100
Bicycling 6 mph (9.7 km/h)	65
Bicycling 12 mph (19 km/h)	100
Tennis, singles	100
Jogging 5.5 mph (8.9 km/h)	160
Jumping rope	160
Cross-country skiing	160

Walking is "just what the doctor ordered" for many people. It's readily available, affordable, usually safe, and requires little instruction. If it's too hot, too cold, or rainy outside, you can do it in a mall, gymnasium, or health club.

Another option is instructional exercise DVDs, often featuring either a celebrity or prominent fitness trainer. Many of these programs require only a pair of sneakers and loose clothing. Others include the option of using inexpensive equipment, such as light hand-held weights.

Another fun option for indoor aerobic exercise is Dance Dance Revolution by Konami. Perhaps you've seen a version of this video game in an arcade. You must use a video game console, such as a PlayStation or Xbox, and the Dance Dance Revolution Controller along with your TV screen. The controller is a

32 inch by 36 inch (81 x 91 cm) floor pad partitioned into several large squares. The TV screen shows you which squares to step on in sequence as the music plays, and you rack up points for accurate timing and foot placement. If you enjoy moving to music, it's more fun than I can describe.

The latest indoor computerized exercise gadgets are the Kinect for Microsoft's Xbox 360, the PlayStation Move, and Wii Fit. Check'em out.

Of late, I've been thinking that exercise isn't really supposed to be fun or enjoyable. If it is, that's just icing on the cake. Maybe exercise is just a chore you need to do for your own good, an investment in quality of life and longevity. Check out this interesting essay by Ken Hutchins on this concept: http://efficientexercise.com/downloads/exercise_vs _recreation.pdf
(Hat tip to Skyler Tanner at http://skylertanner.com/).

MAKE IT A HABIT

The main objective at this point is to make regular physical activity a habit. Establishment of a habit requires frequent repetition over at least two or three months, regardless of the weather, whether you feel like it or not. Over time the chosen activity becomes part of your identity.

PRACTICAL POINTS

To avoid injury and burn out, begin your exercise program slowly and increase the intensity of your effort only every two or three weeks. Your body needs time to adjust to its new workload, but it will indeed adjust. Enhance your enjoyment with proper attire, equipment, and instruction, if needed. Use a portable radio or digital music system like an iPod or Zune if you tend to get bored exercising.

The "buddy system" works well for many of my patients: agree with a friend that you'll meet regularly for walking, jogging, whatever. If you know your buddy is counting on you to show up at the park at 7 a.m., it may be just the motivation you need to get you out of bed. Others just can't handle such regimentation and enjoy the flexibility and independence of solitary activity.

If you like to socialize, join a health club or sports team. Large cities have organized clubs that promote a wide range of physical activities. Find your niche.

Don't be afraid to try something new. Expect some disappointment and failed experiments. Learn and grow from adversity and failure. Put a lot of thought into your choice of activity. Avoid built-in barriers. If you live in Florida you won't have much opportunity for cross-country skiing. If joining a health club is a financial strain, walk instead. Perhaps pick different activities for cold and warm weather. Or do several types of exercise to avoid boredom.

In summary, formation of the exercise habit requires forethought, repetition, and commitment. You must schedule time for physical activity. Make it a priority. Hundreds of my couch potato patients have done it, and I'm sure you can, too. I've seen 40-year-old unathletic, uncoordinated barnacles start exercising and run marathons two years later.

MEDICAL CLEARANCE

To protect you from injury, I recommend that you obtain "medical clearance" from a personal physician before starting an exercise program. A physician is in the best position to determine if your plans are safe for you, thereby avoiding complications such as injury and death. Nevertheless, most adults can start a moderate-intensity exercise program with little risk. An example of moderate intensity would be walking briskly (3–4 mph or 4.8–6.4 km/h) for 30 minutes daily.

Men over 40 and women over 50 who anticipate a more vigorous program should consult a physician to ensure safety. The physician may well recommend diagnostic blood work, an electrocardiogram (heart electrical tracing), and an exercise stress test (often on a treadmill). The goal is not to generate fees for the doctor, but to find the occasional person for whom exercise will be dangerous, if not fatal. Those who drop dead at the start of a vigorous exercise program often have an undiagnosed heart condition, such as blockages in the arteries that supply the heart muscle. The doctor will also look for other dangerous undiagnosed "silent" conditions, such as leaky heart valves, hereditary heart conditions, aneurysms, extremely high blood pressure, and severe diabetes.

Regardless of age, other folks who may benefit from a medical consultation before starting an exercise program include those with known high blood pressure, high cholesterol, joint problems (e.g., arthritis, degenerated discs), neurologic problems, poor circulation, diabetes, lung disease, or any other significant chronic medical condition. Also be sure to check with a doctor first if you've been experiencing chest pains, palpitations, dizziness, fainting spells, headaches, frequent urination, or any unusual symptoms (particularly during exertion).

Physicians, physiatrists, physical therapists, and exercise physiologists can also be helpful in design of a safe, effective exercise program for those with established chronic medical conditions.

GETTING STARTED

I've had otherwise healthy overweight patients so "out of shape" that walking 20 yards (18 meters) to the mailbox was a real chore. They were tired and panting when they got to the mailbox and had to rest a bit before returning to the house. These folks are habitually sedentary and dramatically over-weight. But you need not feel too sorry for them. After starting and maintaining an exercise program, these unfit people achieve the greatest degree of im-provement in fitness level. They make more progress, and faster, than those who begin with a greater level of fitness.

The way to achieve aerobic fitness is to regularly challenge your large muscles to perform sustained physical activity. "Regularly" means at least three days a week, if not daily. I do recommend at least one day of rest weekly.

Left alone, your muscles don't want to do much other than just get you through your day comforta-bly, without effort, aching, or cramps. You must challenge them to do more, work a bit harder, tole-rate a little aching. You will know you are challeng-ing them during exercise when you perceive that mild to moderate effort is required to keep the activ-ity going. You should be mildly short of breath, per-haps even perspiring lightly, yet still able to converse. "Sustained" physical activity means at least 30 minutes in a day. Most people find it a better use of their time to exercise for 30 minutes continuously rather than break it up into five or 10 minutes here and there.

If you're starting out in poor shape, you won't be able to do 30 minutes of any exercise without adverse effects. Don't even try. The worst thing you could do at this point is injure yourself or have such a horrible experience that you give up entirely. Thirty minutes of almost daily activity is your goal to achieve over the next four to 12 months. Moderate to high levels of fitness will take you six to 24 months. The most important thing when getting started is to exercise at least a little, five to 10 minutes, on most days of the week. And don't overdo it in terms of intensity. Start low, go slow. After three months, exercise will be a habit. Prolongation of your exercise sessions will be easy as your amazing body responds gradually to the workload through the process called physical conditioning.

If walking 30 minutes daily is too hard for you at first, try walking just an extra 10 or 20 minutes daily. If you can do that but it's a bit of a strain, gradually (every two weeks) increase your walking time by five minutes daily until you're up to 30 minutes. Average walking pace is 2 mph (3.2 km/h). Once you can comfortably handle 30 minutes daily, the next step is to increase your walking pace to 3 or 4 mph (4.8–6.4 km/h) for the entire 30 minutes. Four mph (6.4 km/h) is definitely a brisk walk. It's difficult for many people to sustain over 30 minutes until they work up to it gradually. This is often done by walking at two paces, normal and brisk, during an exercise session. You might walk five minutes at normal pace, then five minutes briskly, alternating every five minutes until the session is over. Every two to four weeks, you can increase the minutes of brisk pace and taper off the normal pace. You're able to do this easily because your level of fitness is increasing.

I'm asking you to walk briskly (3–4 mph or 4.8–6.4 km/h) for 30 minutes most days of the week. This brisk pace burns roughly 200 calories per session, in case you're wondering. If you eat a 400-calorie muffin, it provides enough energy for a one-hour brisk walk. If you don't burn the muffin calories as exercise or basal metabolism, they'll turn into body fat. (But you're not eating muffins anymore, are you?!)

If you prefer physical activity other than walking, the general rule is to start slowly and gradually increase your effort (intensity) until you're up to about 30 minutes of moderate-intensity exercise most days of the week. Start low, go slow.

IF YOU ARE MARKEDLY OBESE

The more overweight you are, the harder it will be to exercise. At some point even light exercise becomes impossible. A 280-pound (127 kg) woman or 360-pound (164 kg) man isn't going to be able to jog around the block, much less run a marathon. An actual "exercise program" probably won't be possible until some weight is lost simply through very-low-carb eating, calorie restriction, or bariatric surgery. The initial exercise goal for you may just be to get moving through activities of daily living and perhaps brief walks, and calisthenics while sitting in a chair.

Markedly obese people who aren't up to the aforementioned extreme weights can usually tolerate a low-intensity physical activity program. Many obese people are lugging around 70 to 90 pounds (32 to 41 kg) of excess weight. This weight burden causes dramatic breathlessness and fatigue upon exertion, and makes the joints and muscles more susceptible to aching and injury. If you're skinny, just imagine trying to walk or run a mile carrying a standard five-gallon (19 liter) water cooler bottle, which weighs only 43 pounds (19.5 kg) when full. The burden of excess fat makes it quite difficult to exercise.

If you're markedly obese, several tricks will enhance your exercise success. I want you to avoid injury, frustration, and burn out. Start with light activity for only 10 or 15 minutes, gradually increase session length (e.g., by two to four minutes every two to four weeks) and increase exercise intensity only after several months. Your joints and muscles may appreciate easy, low-impact exercises such as stationary cycling, walking, swimming, pool calisthenics, and water aerobics. You may also benefit from the advice of a personal fitness trainer arranged through a health club, gym, or YMCA/YWCA. Check out several health clubs before you join. Some of them are primarily meat markets for beautiful slender yuppies. You may feel more comfortable in a gym that welcomes and caters to overweight people. Hospitals are increasingly developing fitness centers with obese orthopedic, heart, and diabetic patients in mind.

PEDOMETERS

A pedometer attached to your waistband may help motivate you by tracking total step count, distance traveled, and calories burned. Reliable pedometers cost $20 to $35 (USD) and are available at sporting goods stores, sports shoe stores, and via the Internet.

Good pedometers are the Omron HJ 112, the Accusplit AE 170 XLG, the Omron HIP (HJ 150), and the Omron HJ-303

Sedentary people walk 2,000–4,000 steps daily as they go about their lives. Your goal now is 8,000–10,000 daily steps. Ten-thousand steps covers about 5 miles (8 kilometers).

A high-tech alternative to a pedometer is Nike+ (Nike Plus), which is geared more toward runners.

TARGET HEART RATE

One rough way to gauge whether you're working hard enough during exercise is to monitor your heart rate, also known as pulse. Subtract your age from 220. The result is your theoretical maximum heart rate in beats per minute. Your heart rate goal, or target, during sustained aerobic exercise is a pulse that is 60 to 80% of your theoretical maximum pulse. For example: maximum heart rate for a 40-year-old is 180 (220 - 40 = 180), so the target heart rate zone during exercise is between 108 and 144 (60 to 80% of 180). Exceeding the upper end of the target zone is usually too uncomfortable to be sustainable. Exercise heart rates below the target zone suggest you're not working hard enough to reap the full long-term benefits of aerobic exercise.

Here's how to determine your pulse. After five or 10 minutes of exercise, stop moving and place the tips of your first two fingers lightly over the pulse spot inside your wrist just below the base of your thumb. Count the pulsations for 15 seconds and multiply the number by four. The result is your pulse or heart rate. It will take some practice to find those pulsations coming from your radial artery. If you can't find it, ask a nurse or doctor for help.

Like all rules-of-thumb, this target heart rate zone isn't always an accurate gauge of cardiovascular workout intensity. For instance, it's of very little use in people taking drugs called beta blockers, which keep a lid on heart rate.

As you become more fit, you'll notice that you have to work harder to get your heart rate up to a certain level. This is a sure sign that your heart and muscles are responding to your challenge. You may also want to monitor your resting heart rate taken in the morning before you get out of bed. Unfit, sedentary people have resting pulses of 60 to 90. Athletes are more often in the 40s or low 50s. Their hearts have become more efficient and just don't need to beat as often to get the job done.

As you become more fit, you'll also notice that you have more energy overall and it's easier to move about and handle physical workloads. You'll feel more relaxed and have a sense of accomplishment. Expect these benefits eight to 12 weeks after starting a regular exercise program.

EXERCISE WITH JOINT AND BACK PAIN

Painful lower limb joints and chronic or recurrent back pain are an exercise barrier to many people. Those affected should consult a physician for diagnosis, treatment, and advice on appropriate physical activity. If the physician isn't sure about an exercise prescription, consultation with an orthopedist, physiatrist, or physical therapist should be helpful. Generally, weight-bearing on bad joints should be minimized by doing pool calisthenics, stationary cycling, swimming, etc. Use your imagination. Particularly bothersome joints may not tolerate exercise, if ever, until weight is lost by other methods, such as very-low-carb eating. Light to moderate exercise actually reduces the pain and disability of knee degenerative arthritis. The effect is modest and comes with a small risk of injury such as bone fracture, cartilage tears, arthritis flare, and soft tissue strain.

SUMMARY

Again, the goal is 30 minutes of brisk walking most days of the week, plus strength training three days a week. Walking faster or longer, and more vigorous types of exercise, might help you lose weight faster and achieve higher levels of fitness. But committing much more time and energy to exercise just isn't going to happen for many folks. Fortunately, most of the general health benefits of an active lifestyle are gained by a simple 30-minute daily brisk walk or similar aerobic exercise.

You may still be able to control your weight even if you don't exercise, particularly if you avoid the fattening carbohydrates like concentrated sugars and refined starches.

If you can't manage regular physical activity during your period of weight loss, at least give it another chance as you move into your maintenance-of-weight-loss phase. Regular exercise is the single best predictor of successful long-term weight management.

Exercise may not be easy, it may not be popular, it may not be what you want to hear, but it's the right thing to do.

KEY POINTS

- Lack of regular exercise causes preventable deaths.
- Increasing your level of fitness can reduce your risk of death from cardiovascular disease and cancer.
- Exercise turns body fat into weightless energy, unless you eat too much.
- Once you lose your excess weight, regular exercise will greatly enhance your success in keeping the weight off.
- Exercise is a demonstrable fountain of youth.

10
Long-Term Maintenance and Prevention of Weight Regain

Reaccumulation of lost body fat is the most problematic area in the field of weight management. You may have heard that "diets don't work," but they do. Many different programs work short-term, if "work" is defined as loss of five, 10, or more pounds (two, four, or more kg) while you adhere to the program for several weeks or months. The problem is that the lost pounds usually return. You get bored with the diet, or your will-power flags, or the diet simply stops working, the transition from weight loss to maintenance is unclear, you just feel too bad to go on, you lose your commitment, you take a job as a taste tester for Baskin-Robbins Ice Cream, or whatever.

Most diets ultimately fail in the long run simply because people go back to their old habits.

FINALLY AT GOAL WEIGHT

For purposes of further discussion, I'll assume that you've already lost weight down to your goal and now must focus on staying thereabouts from here on out.

Finally down to your goal! A grand accomplishment! You've got a new wardrobe, or the old clothes fit again. You have more energy and feel younger. Maybe you cured or improved some health problems. Perhaps you're getting more attention from the opposite sex.

The scientific name for humans is *Homo sapiens*. Sapiens is from the Latin sapere, which means "to be wise." Wisdom is the ability to make correct judgments and decisions. Undoubtedly, your success at weight loss required correct judgments and decisions. You're not done yet. You'll need sustained wisdom to avoid weight regain.

Be wise about this especially: you can never again eat all you want, whatever you want, whenever you want, over sustained periods of time.

I'm sorry. But somebody has to tell you the truth.

Now that you've reached your goal weight, you must restrain yourself on a daily basis. Think about it. You became overweight because you didn't watch what you ate. Inadequate exercise may well have contributed, too. You can't go back to your old ways. Reject this advice, and you have a 100 percent chance of regaining your lost weight.

Now that you're at your goal weight and want to stay there, you can add some calories back into the energy balance equation. Add the calories by eating more food, exercising less, or a combination of the two. But if you add back too many calories, you'll regain weight. Carbohydrate calories are particularly effective at packing the fat back on, because they stimulate release of the fat-building hormone, insulin. The fattening carbohydrates typically are concentrated sugars and refined starches.

TRANSITION TO MAINTENANCE PHASE: THE LOW-CARB MEDITERRANEAN DIET

I'll assume readers of this section have been following the Ketogenic Mediterranean Diet (KMD) for at least a couple weeks, if not for several months or more. I recommend at least 8–12 weeks.

At this point you're ready for a change either because you've reached your weight-loss goal or you want a greater variety of carbohydrates (carbs). Stay familiar with the KMD because it's the foundation for everything that will follow. You're not really done with it; you're adding to it, moving from a very-low-carb diet to the Low-Carb Mediterranean Diet.

The Low-Carb Mediterranean Diet (LCMD) loosens up on food restrictions and introduces additional carbohydrates as long as weight management doesn't deteriorate.

Perhaps you've been losing weight steadily with the KMD and are not yet at your goal weight but crave more food variety. Many continue to lose excess weight with the Low-Carb Mediterranean Diet, although it tends to be easier with the KMD. If weight loss stalls, just return to the KMD.

Alternatively, perhaps you're simply interested in eating more of the plant-based foods linked to the health benefits of the traditional Mediterranean diet.

The KMD may be perfectly healthy long-term; we just don't know for sure. I think it is. On the other hand, we have at least some evidence that additional carbohydrates, as in the Low-Carb Mediterranean Diet, may be even healthier. For example, some scientific studies link higher fruit and vegetable consumption with lower rates of cancer, stroke, and coronary heart disease. (Other studies find no benefit.) Whole grain consumption is associated with lower rates of cardiovascular disease, including heart attacks and strokes. Legumes (such as beans and peas) are a great source of fiber to counteract the constipation common with very-low-carb diets like the KMD. Additional fruits and vegetables might contribute to longevity, prevent dementia, and help preserve vision by preventing macular degeneration.

And some added carbohydrates may just plain taste good!

My primary goal with the KMD and LCMD is to reap the health benefits of a Mediterranean style diet while not allowing too many fattening carbs that sabotage weight-management efforts.

OVERVIEW OF THE LOW-CARB MEDITERRANEAN DIET

You've been eating 20 to 30 grams of digestible carbohydrate daily on the KMD. Now you're going to increase to 40–100 grams daily, gradually adding carbs that may have beneficial effects on health and longevity. Adding excessive carbs will lead inevitably to regain of lost weight, or a stall in weight-loss progress.

Also note that excessive consumption of easily digested carbs is linked to future diabetes, heart disease, and gallbladder disease, at least in women. So we may as well aim for reasonable carb restriction.

If you're not at your goal weight already, adding too many carb grams now will impair your ability to convert your body fat into energy. Eat too many carbs, and your body will use them for the energy it needs rather than your body's fat. You may well continue to lose weight eating 40, 60, or 100 grams a day, but maybe not. Remember, the typical American adult eats about 275 grams of carb daily, and two thirds of us are overweight or obese.

LET'S GET STARTED ON LCMD!

So, what healthy carbs are we going to add to the Ketogenic Mediterranean Diet, transforming it into the Low-Carb Mediterranean Diet? Fruits, more vegetables (including starchy ones), legumes, yogurt and other dairy products, and whole grains.

To avoid carb overdose and loss of weight control, we're adding back carbs incrementally and slowly.

I've divided the new carbohydrates into groups and specified a serving size for each source of carbs. Each serving has about 7.5 grams of digestible carbohydrate. See Table 9.1.

Table 9.1 Carb Groups and Serving Sizes
for the Low-Carb Mediterranean Diet

(Each serving has about 7.5 grams of digestible carbohy-drate.)

Fruits

apple, a third of medium-sized one (54 g)
banana, one third (39 g)
peach, ½ of medium (75 g)
strawberry halves, two thirds of a cup (75 g)
blueberries, ½ cup (75 g)
raspberries, 1 cup (123 g)
blackberries, 1 cup (144 g)
cantaloupe, ½ cup cubes (80 g)
honeydew, 1 cup of cubes (85 g)
date, medjool, ½ date (12 g)
orange, navel, ½ (70 g)
pear, a third of medium-sized one (60 g)
pomegranate, ¼ of 4" (10 cm) diameter fruit (70g)
tangerine, ½ (44 g)
grapefruit, ½ (61 g)
cherries, sweet, raw, a third of a cup (45 g)
grapes, a third of a cup (50 g)
raisins, seedless, 20 (9 g)
nectarine, medium, ½ (70 g)
mango, slices, a third of a cup (55 g)
pineapple, raw chunks, a third of a cup (55g)
lime/lemon juice, raw, 2 limes or lemons (88 g)
watermelon, diced, two thirds of a cup (100 g)

Vegetables and Fruits

potato, white, raw, flesh and skin,
     ¼ of medium potato (53 g)
corn, canned, drained, ¼ cup (41g)
carrots, raw, strips or slices, ¾ cup (92 g)

sweet potato, raw, a third of 5 inch-long (13 cm)
    tater (45 g)
beets, canned, drained solids, ¾ cup slices (130 g)
peas, green, canned or frozen, ½ cup (67 g)
spaghetti squash, cooked, 1 cup (155 g)
KMD mixed veggies, 7 oz (200 g)

Legumes

peas, split, mature seeds, cooked/boiled,
    ¼ cup (49 g)
peas, black-eyed (cowpeas), canned, ¼ cup (60 g)
soybeans, mature seeds, roasted, 1.5 oz (42 g)
soybeans, mature seeds, cooked/boiled,
    1 cup (170 g)
beans, mature seeds, cooked/boiled, ¼ cup (43 g)
    (beans = black, kidney, navy, pinto, white, fava,
    chickpeas/garbanzo)

Yogurt and Milk Products

yogurt, plain whole milk, ½ cup
milk, whole, ½ cup
milk, 1% milk fat, ½ cup
Fage Greek, "total 2%", ½ cup (get full-fat version
    if available)
Voskos plain original Greek yogurt, ½ cup

Grains

bread, whole wheat, ½ slice (15 g)
bread, Ezekiel 4:19, ½ slice
pasta, 100% whole grain, dry, 12 g
Ry-Krisp crackers, 4.5 x 2.5" (11 x 6 cm) (11 g)
Triscuit crackers x 3 (14 g)
cracker, whole wheat, 14 g
tortilla (Mission), 8" (20 cm) whole grain,

a third of a tortilla (16 g)
oats, dry whole grain, a third of a cup uncooked
  (13 g)
oats, steel-cut, uncooked, 1.3 tbsp (13 g)
rice, brown, cooked, 3 tbsp
quinoa, cooked, 3 tbsp (35 g)
barley, pearled, cooked, 3 tbsp (30g)
shredded wheat, plain, sugar-free (11 g)
cereal, FiberOne, original, plain,
  a third of a cup or 5 tbsp (75 ml)
Kellogg's All-Bran original or
  All-Bran Bran Buds, ¼ cup (15 g)

Table 9.1 Carb Groups and Serving Sizes
for the Low-Carb Mediterranean Diet

What you do next is add one daily carb serving from
the list of Carb Groups and Serving Sizes in Table
9.1 and see what happens with your weight over the
next week. This is not one carb serving on Monday,
two on Tuesday, three on Wednesday, etc. It's seven
new carb servings per week, one on each day.

Essentially, you still eat the Ketogenic Mediterranean Diet but are adding a daily carb serving. If you
have unwanted weight gain, or your weight loss
progress stalls, you've added too many carbs and
must cut back, or try different carb sources.

On the other hand, if you handled the extra carb
serving without trouble for a week, you may add one
more daily carb serving. Monitor your progress for
another week.

If you're handling those carbs, you may increase by
one additional carb serving every week. You've added too much carb if you gain unwanted weight, or
your weight loss progress stalls. Then you must cut

back or try different carbs, especially different carb groups.

Weigh yourself daily during the first two months of your maintenance phase. After that, weigh at least weekly. Daily weights will remind you how hard you worked to achieve your goal. When you look now at a brownie, candy bar, or piece of pie, you ask yourself, "Do I really want to walk an extra hour or jog an extra three miles today to burn off those calories?" If so, enjoy. Otherwise, forego the unneeded calories.

Many people who have weight management problems will not be able to increase carbs to more than six additional daily servings. But that's OK because you don't necessarily need more carbs for a long and healthy life. For many folks, additional carbs are unhealthy.

By the way, if you wish to cut back on your animal protein consumption at this point, feel free. It's your choice. I'd continue to eat cold-water fatty fish at least two or three times weekly, along with the usual olive oil and nuts.

Are you with me so far?

WHICH CARBS TO ADD

OK, so you're going to add some carbs to your diet, but which ones? For the potential health benefits, I'd add carbs in this order:
- fruits
- vegetables
- whole grains
- legumes
- yogurt and other dairy products

This is just a loose guideline, not a commandment. I suggest everyone eventually add one or two servings of fruit daily, classic fruits rather than technical fruits like tomato and avocado already on the KMD. Legumes, yogurt, and other dairy products are listed after fruits and veggies because the evidence in favor of their long-term health benefits isn't as strong. Eating a couple servings of whole grain daily is fairly consistently linked to a reduced risk of heart disease.

Yogurt deserves special mention because it's a component of the traditional doctor-recommended Mediterranean diet. It's a great source of calcium, a critical mineral for healthy bones, nerves, and muscles. Does it have anything special you couldn't get elsewhere? Probably not.

Now you're ready to enhance the KMD with an extra carb serving daily. Why not start with a fruit? Choose a variety of items within any given carb group, and try eventually to eat from multiple carb groups. Variety ensures you get adequate vitamins, minerals, and phytonutrients.

Nevertheless, just to be sure, continue your supplements as on the KMD. If you're sick of taking them, drop the calcium first, potassium second, magnesium third, and finally the multivitamin/multimineral. Wait a couple weeks between each discontinuation, and monitor how you feel. Any weakness? Fatigue? Muscle cramps? Restart the dropped supplement and see if it resolves the issue.

Once your total daily digestible carb grams are up in the 60–100 g range, you have my blessing to start dropping some of the supplements you've been taking, one supplement every week or two as above.

Vitamin D is special. If you don't get much sun exposure, I'd continue to take 1,000 IU daily, indefinitely. See what your own doctor thinks. You might also benefit from ongoing daily supplementation with a multivitamin.

FOR YOUR CONVENIENCE ...

You can print a copy of the Carb Groups and Serving Sizes from this web page:
http://advancedmediterraneandiet.com/printabledocuments.html
You'll also find a grocery shopping list for the both the KMD and LCMD at the same page.

Welcome to the Low-Carb Mediterranean Diet!

WHAT IF I GAIN A LITTLE WEIGHT BACK?

Be aware that you might regain five or 10 pounds (two to four kg) of fat now and then. You probably will. It's not the end of the world. It's human nature. You're not a failure; you're human. But draw the line and get back on the old KMD for one or two months.

Analyze and learn from the episode. Why did it happen? Slipping back into your old ways? Slacking off on exercise? Too many special occasion feasts? Allowing junk food with fattening carbs back into the house?

It's OK to overindulge in food infrequently (10–12 times per year), on special occasions such as birthdays, wedding anniversaries, holidays. But you must counteract the extra calories by cutting down intake or by exercising more, either before or after the feast.

TWO SECRETS TO KEEPING THE WEIGHT OFF

The true measure of a successful weight management program is not simply how much weight is lost, but whether the lost weight stays lost over the long run. What distinguishes weight losers who keep the weight off from those who gain it back? Two factors, mostly:

1. Restrained eating
2. Regular physical activity

"Successful losers" apply self-restraint on an almost daily basis, avoiding food they know will lead to weight regain. They limit how much they eat. They consciously choose not to return to their old eating habits, despite urges to the contrary.

The other glaring difference is that, compared to regainers, the successful losers are physically active. Oftentimes, they exercised while losing weight, and almost always continue to exercise in the maintenance phase of their program. This is true in at least eight out of 10 cases. It's clear that regular exercise isn't always needed, but it dramatically increases your chances of long-term success.

THE PAYOFF

Congratulations, in advance perhaps, on accomplishing a worthwhile, difficult goal through Mediterranean-style eating! You now know how your body uses various nutrients and energy, and how to apply that knowledge to optimize your health and longevity. You now know that excess body fat and certain nutrients contribute to disease. Other specific nutrients promote health. You now know how to build a social support system to assist in your weight control endeavor. This knowledge base motivated you to persevere when you were tempted to abandon the effort. Your careful attention to the daily logs has confirmed and reinforced your discipline. The transformation to your slimmer body required commitment and willpower, which you may have thought at one time were in short supply. You no longer live to eat, but eat to live.

Now, be wise and do something great for those around you with your renewed vigor and longer life.

KEY POINTS

- Get real about weight gain. You can never again eat all you want, whenever you want, over sustained periods of time.
- "Successful losers" who don't regain the weight share two characteristics: 1) restrained eating habits, and 2) regular physical activity.
- Most diets ultimately fail in the long run simply because people go back to their old habits. If you return to what you always did, you'll keep getting what you always got: gradual weight gain.
- In transitioning from the Ketogenic Mediterranean Diet to the Low-Carb Mediterranean Diet, carbohydrates must be added slowly and incrementally.

- Many people will not be successful at weight management if they eat over 80–100 grams of digestible carbohydrates daily.
- Continue careful monitoring of your food intake and exercise during the first two months of your maintenance phase.
- Weigh yourself daily during the first two months of your maintenance phase. After that, weigh at least weekly for the rest of your life.
- You might regain five or 10 pounds (two or four kg) now and then. If so, simply return to your previously successful weight-loss diet for one to two months. No big deal.

RECOMMENDED FURTHER READING

Books

Bittman, Mark. *How to Cook Everything: 2,000 Simple Recipes for Great Food*. Wiley, 2008.

Cloutier, Marissa and Adamson, Eve. *The Mediterranean Diet* (revised and updated). Avon Books, 2004.

Cook's Illustrated. *The New Best Recipes*. America's Test Kitchen, 2004.

Crocker, Betty. *Betty Crocker Cookbook: 1500 Recipes for the Way You Cook Today*. Betty Crocker, 2011.

Eloff, Jennifer; Emmerich, Maria; Ketchum, Carolyn; Marshall, Lisa; and Altena, Kent. *Low-Carbing Among Friends,* Volume 1. Eureka Publishing, 2011.

Jenkins, Nancy Harmon. *The New Mediterranean Diet Cookbook: A Delicious Alternative for Lifelong Health*. Bantam, 2008.

Rombauer, Irma S.; Becker, Marion Rombauer; and Becker, Ethan. *Joy of Cooking: 75th Anniversary Edition*. Scribner, 2006

Taubes, Gary. *Why We Get Fat: And What to Do About It*. Knopf, 2011.

Volek, Jeff and Phinney, Stephen. *The Art and Science of Low Carbohydrate Living: An Expert Guide to Making the Life-Saving Benefits of Carbohydrate Restriction Sustainable and Enjoyable*. Beyond Obesity LLC, 2011.

Westman, Eric; Phinney, Stephen; and Volek, Jeff. *The New Atkins for a New You: The Ultimate Diet for Shedding Weight and Feeling Great*. Fireside, 2010.

Whitney, Eleanor Noss and Rolfes, Sharon Rady. *Understanding Nutrition* (10th edition). Wadsworth Publishing Company, 2010.

Internet

About.com: Low Carb Diets. Guide: Laura Dolson.
http://lowcarbdiets.about.com/

Recommended Further Reading

All Day I Dream About Food (low-carb recipes by Carolyn)
http://dreamaboutfood.blogspot.com/

Allrecipes.com
http://www.allrecipes.com
"Devoted to a community of home cooks," this site has over
30,000 free recipes with detailed nutritional analysis, including
calories per serving. Numerous Mediterranean-style dishes (enter
search word "Mediterranean").

Clifford A. Wright
http://www.cliffordawright.com
This cook and writer specializes in regional cuisines of the Mediterranean region, with emphasis on culinary history. You'll find
some recipes here along with historical articles and numerous
helpful Internet links.

DARdreams (low-carb recipes)
http://dardreams.wordpress.com/

Fat Head by Tom Naughton (low-carb lifestyle)
http://www.fathead-movie.com/

Healthy Low-Carb Living by Amy Dungan
http://healthylowcarbliving.com/

Hold the Toast! by Dana Carpender (low-carb lifestyle)
http://holdthetoast.com/

Jimmy Moore's Livin' La Vida Low Carb Blog (renowned low-carb
advocate)
http://livinlavidalowcarb.com/blog/

Oldways Preservation and Exchange Trust
http://www.oldwayspt.org
This nonprofit "food issues think tank" facilitates the translation
of nutrition science into practical healthy eating patterns, including the traditional Mediterranean diet.

Physical Activity for Everyone
http://www.cdc.gov/nccdphp/dnpa/physical/

Shape Up America!
http://www.shapeup.org
"Founded in 1994, Shape Up America! is a 501(c)3
not-for-profit organization committed to raising awareness of
obesity as a health issue and to providing responsible information on healthy weight management."

Splendid Low-Carbing by Jennifer Eloff (low-carb recipes)
http://low-carb-news.blogspot.com/

The Blog of Michael R. Eades, M.D. (low-carb advocate and co-author of *Protein Power*)
http://proteinpower.com/drmike/

Weight-Control Information Network
http://www.win.niddk.nih.gov/index.htm
A service of the (U.S.) National Institute of Diabetes and Digestive and Kidney Diseases. Information for the public and healthcare professionals on obesity, weight control, related nutritional matters, and physical activity.

SELECTED REFERENCES BY TOPIC

Topics

Dietary Fat Doesn't Cause Heart and Vascular
Disease
Superior Effectiveness of Low-Carb Dieting

You can read most of these articles or their abstracts online at
the publishing journal's website.

Dietary Fat Doesn't Cause Heart and Vascular Disease

Siri-Tarino, Patty, et al. Meta-analysis of prospective cohort studies evaluating the association of saturated fat with cardiovascular disease. *American Journal of Clinical Nutrition,*
January 13, 2010. doi:10.3945/ajcn.2009.27725

Skeaff, C. Murray and Miller, Jody. Dietary fat and coronary
heart disease: Summary of evidence from prospective cohort
and randomised controlled trials. *Annals of Nutrition and
Metabolism,* 55 (2009): 173–201.

Halton, Thomas, et al. Low-carbohydrate-diet score and the risk
of coronary heart disease in women. *New England Journal of
Medicine,* 355 (2006): 1,991–2,002.

German, J. Bruce, and Dillard, Cora J. Saturated fats: What
dietary intake? *American Journal of Clinical Nutrition,* 80
(2004): 550–559.

Ravnskov, U. The questionable role of saturated and
polyunsaturated fatty acids in cardiovascular disease. *Journal of Clinical Epidemiology,* 51 (1998): 443–460.

Ravsnskov, U. Hypothesis out-of-date. The diet-heart idea. *Journal of Clinical Epidemiology,* 55 (2002): 1,057–1,063.

Ravnskov, U, et al. Studies of dietary fat and heart disease.
Science, 295 (2002): 1,464-1,465.

Taubes, G. The soft science of dietary fat. *Science,* 291 (2001):
2,535–2,541.

Zarraga, Ignatius, and Schwartz, Ernst. Impact of dietary patterns and interventions on cardiovascular health. *Circulation*, 114 (2006): 961–973.

Mente, Andrew, et al. A Systematic Review of the Evidence Supporting a Causal Link Between Dietary Factors and Coronary Heart Disease. *Archives of Internal Medicine*, 169 (2009): 659–669.

Parikh, Parin, et al. Diets and cardiovascular disease: an evidence-based assessment. *Journal of the American College of Cardiology*, 45 (2005): 1,379–1,387.

Hooper, L., et al. Dietary fat intake and prevention of cardiovascular disease: systematic review. *British Medical Journal*, 322 (2001): 757-763.

Weinberg, W.C. The Diet-Heart Hypothesis: a critique. *Journal of the American College of Cardiology*, 43 (2004): 731–733.

Mozaffarian, Darius, et al. Dietary fats, carbohydrate, and progression of coronary atherosclerosis in postmenopausal women. *American Journal of Clinical Nutrition*, 80 (2004): 1,175–1,184.

Knopp, Robert and Retzlaff, Barbara. Saturated fat prevents coronary artery disease? An American paradox. *American Journal of Clinical Nutrition*, 80 (2004): 1,102–1,103.

Yusuf, S., et al. Effect of potentially modifiable risk factors associated with myocardial infarction in 52 countries (the INTERHEART study): case-control study. *Lancet*, 364 (2004): 937–952. (ApoB/ApoA1 ratio was a risk factor for heart attack, so dietary saturated fat may play a role if it affects this ratio.)

Hu, Frank. Diet and cardiovascular disease prevention: The need for a paradigm shift. *Journal of the American College of Cardiology*, 50 (2007): 22–24.

Oh, K., et al. Dietary fat intake and risk of coronary heart disease in women: 20 years of follow-up of the Nurses' Health Study. *American Journal of Epidemiology*, 161 (2005): 672–679.

Superior Effectiveness of Low-Carb Dieting

Brehm, B.J., et al. A randomized trial comparing a very low carbohydrate diet and a calorie-restricted low fat diet on body weight and cardiovascular risk factors in healthy women. Journal *of Clinical Endocrinology and Metabolism*, 88 (2003): 1,617–1,623.

Samaha, F.F., et al. A low-carbohydrate as compared with a low-fat diet in severe obesity. *New England Journal of Medicine*, 348 (2003): 2,074–2,081.

Sondike, S.B., et al. Effects of a low-carbohydrate diet on weight loss and cardiovascular risk factor in overweight adolescents. *Journal of Pediatrics*, 143 (2003): 253–258.

Aude, Y.W., et al. The National Cholesterol Education Program diet versus a diet lower in carbohydrates and higher in protein and monounsaturated fat. A randomized trial. *Archives of Internal Medicine*, 164 (2004): 2,141–2,146.

Volek, J.S., et al. Comparison of energy-restricted very low-carbohydrate and low-fat diets on weight loss and body composition in overweight men and women. *Nutrition & Metabolism*, 1 (2004), 1:13.

Yancy, W.S. Jr, et al. A low-carbohydrate, ketogenic diet versus a low-fat diet to treat obesity and hyperlipidemia. A randomized, controlled trial. *Annals of Internal Medicine*, 140 (2004): 769–777.

Nichols-Richardsson, S.M., et al. Perceived hunger is lower and weight loss is greater in overweight premenopausal women consuming a low-carbohydrate/high- protein versus high-carbohydrate/low-fat diet. *Journal of the American Dietetic Association*, 105 (205): 1,433–1,437.

Gardner, C.D., et al. Comparison of the Atkins, Zone, Ornish, and Learn diets for change in weight and related risk factors among overweight premenopausal women. The A to Z Weight Loss Study: A randomized trial. *Journal of the American Medical Association*, 297 (2007): 969–977.

Shai, I., et al. Weight loss with a low-carbohydrate, Mediterranean, or low-fat diet. *New England Journal of Medicine*, 359 (2008): 229–241.

Dyson, P.A., et al. A low-carbohydrate diet is more effective in reducing body weight than healthy eating in both diabetic and non-diabetic subjects. *Diabetic Medicine*, 24 (2007): 1,430–1,435.

Krebs, N.F., et al. Efficacy and safety of a high protein, low carbohydrate diet for weight loss in severely obese adolescents. Journal of Pediatrics, 157 (2010): 252–258.

Summer, S.S., et al. Adiponectin changes in relation to the macronutrient composition of a weight-loss diet. *Obesity*, (March 31, 2011). doi: 10.1038/oby.2011.60.

Daly, M.E., et al. Short-term effects of severe dietary carbohydrate-restriction advice in type 2 diabetes. A randomized controlled trial. *Diabetes Medicine*, 23 (2006): 15–20.

Westman, E.C., et al. The effect of a low carbohydrate, ketogenic diet versus a low-glycemic index diet on glycemic control in type 2 diabetes mellitus. *Nutrition and Metabolism*, 5 (2008): 36 (December 19).

RECIPE INDEX

INDEX

Index

About the Author

Dr. Steve Parker is an Internal Medicine specialist with three decades' experience treating people with overweight and obesity, high blood pressure, heart disease, strokes, diabetes, and metabolic syndrome. He's a leading medical expert on the Mediterranean diet. Dr. Parker lives with his wife and children in Scottsdale, Arizona, U.S.A.

30550144R00123

Made in the USA
San Bernardino, CA
17 February 2016